What People

"In a writing style similar to Elizabeth Gilbert's *Eat, Pray, Love*, Michelle reveals her own version of the life story that many of us have experienced on our way to discovering inner peace and inner strength. I laughed out loud and at the same time, her words touched my soul. This is one of the most inspirational and timely books on yoga in the world today. We need this book!"

~ Desiree Rumbaugh, Certified Yoga Teacher and author of *Yoga to the Rescue* DVD

"Michelle's honest, warm and inviting story is a must-read for anyone seeking to find their truth through the practice of yoga. Growing older gracefully is no easy task, and *Finding More on the Mat* reminds us that we are not walking the path alone and that true wisdom and strength can only be found through dedicated efforts over the course of our lives. May this story inspire and bless your efforts."

~ Christina Sell, bestselling author of *Yoga From the Inside Out: Making Peace with Your Body Through Yoga* and *My Body is a Temple: Yoga as a Path to Wholeness*

"Hilarious, poignant, and real, Michelle delivers a down-to-earth account of how yoga touches and transforms us in all aspects of our lives. You won't want to put it down!"

~ Amy Ippoliti, International Yoga Teacher and Earth Advocate

"Michelle can veer from acerbic one-liners to the deepest profundities all while making you feel like her best friend. Read this book! If not for the pure joy of it, then just to get a hit of a fabulous example of a human being."

~ Ross Rayburn, Certified Yoga Teacher

"Reading this wonderful book is much like being in class with Michelle. You will be laughing through your tears all the way to enlightenment! By weaving everyday stories with the ancient teachings, Michelle allows us to absorb a deep lesson about life, love and yoga with grace and laughter."

~ Heather Peterson, West Coast Director, CorePower Yoga

"Memoirs are a dime a dozen today. Then along comes Michelle Marchildon and her amazing *Finding More on the Mat*. Not just a memoir. Not just a book about why you should do yoga and get your health, body and life together. Not just a joy ride if you want to tickle your funny bone. And certainly not just something woven with profound thoughts and wakeups. *Finding More on the Mat* is all those things, and more. It's a true breath of fresh air."

~ Judith Briles, Book Shepherd and author of *The Confidence Factor* and *Show Me About Book Publishing*

Finding More

on the Mat

Finding More
on the Mat

How I Grew Better, Wiser and Stronger through Yoga

Revised Edition

Michelle Berman Marchildon

*Based on the true life experiences
of a recovering corporate executive,
award-winning journalist, yogi, wife, mother
and survivor of fifty years of life.*

HOHM PRESS
Chino Valley, AZ

First Edition: ISBN: 978-0-9848755-0-4
Library of Congress Control Number: 2011945538

Library of Congress Cataloging-in-Publication Data

Marchildon, Michelle Berman.
  Finding more on the mat : how i grew better, wiser and stronger through yoga / Michelle Berman Marchildon. -- Second edition, revised.
    pages cm
  "Based on the true life experiences of a recovering corporate executive, award-winning journalist, yogi, wife, mother and survivor of fifty years of life."
  Includes bibliographical references and index.
  ISBN 978-1-935387-94-7
  1. Yoga. I. Title.
  B132.Y6M2998 2015
  181'.45--dc23
                                        2014042560

Hohm Press
PO Box 4410
Chino Valley, AZ 86323
800-381-2700
www.hohmpress.com

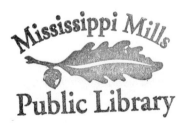

For my children:
always be exactly who you are.

It is better to do your own duty badly,
than to perfectly do another's.
You are safe from harm
when you do what you should be doing.
~ The Bhagavad Gita, 3.35
(Translation by Stephen Mitchell)

If I had known the truth would set me free,
I would have told it much sooner.
~ Michelle Berman Marchildon

Contents

What Is "Something More"?

What are we talking about when we say "more" as yogis?

Certainly *more*, from a yoga perspective, isn't the more that Madison Avenue spends millions of dollars every year to convince us that we need. Certainly, *more* in yoga is not more money, more fame, more beauty, more things, more acquisitions, and so on. And lest you think I am a renunciate or something like that, let's be very clear: I do not think those things are NOT yoga. I just do not think they are the *point* of yoga.

Like so many things in yoga, the concept of *more* is paradoxical. What are we looking for? What is it that we seek? Are we searching outside ourselves? Or do we seek within?

So many times, we find something inside ourselves in yoga that feels like more, or something other and new, and yet it is who we have been all along. But recognizing this quality as our truth, realizing its potential, living from it and being deeply rooted in it, are all different things.

We practice to remind ourselves that we are this something more. We make the connection to our truth as it exists both in potentiality within us and in our moment-to-moment experiences. Seeing our truth and living from it could be the point of our seeking. It could be the point of yoga.

Luckily for us, Michelle found something more on her mat. Her journey from an accidental yogi to a genuinely spiritual being is often hilarious, sometimes poignant, always inspiring and a deeply truthful awakening. Her words are pure joy and a reminder that this thing we seek is closer than we think.

CHRISTINA SELL, author of *Yoga from the Inside Out: Making Peace with Your Body Through Yoga* and *My Body is a Temple: Yoga as a Path to Wholeness*

March 5, 2014

Author's Note to the Second Edition

In yoga, you get a second chance to do the pose.

Although I worked on *Finding More on the Mat* for five years, and lived it for more than fifty, I am grateful to Hohm Press for this second edition and therefore a second chance. Because writing a book is just like yoga.

**You have to be willing to do it over
and over again, until you get it right.**

I call this edition, "What I know now that I wish I knew then." The Universe wants you to experience the good and the bad, the hilarious and the ridiculous, the happy and sad at the same time. I just wish it came with a crystal ball so I would know which people to trust.

This second edition has a new story about an epic fail. I have changed a few of my regrets, and most gratefully, I am able to clarify a few things I originally thought were muddy. Hindsight is the most punishing editor.

"No effort is ever wasted," we learn from the *Bhagavad Gita*, the classic poem about discovering *dharma* that serves as an archetype for *Finding More*. If your practice is not yet perfect, your effort will help you find *more* tomorrow.

This second edition is more precise than the first, but ultimately, it is still just "practice" for living a life better, wiser and stronger than yesterday. I offer it to you to explain that a life well lived, although imperfectly lived, may serve to inspire your path.

MICHELLE MARCHILDON, at her kitchen table in Denver, Colorado. March 5, 2014

Prologue

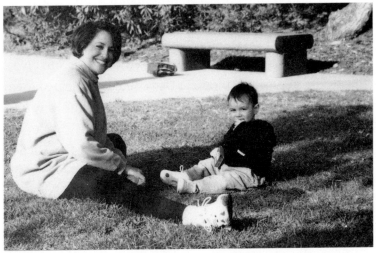

At the beginning of my journey. Above all, yoga made me a better mom.

I came to the mat just before my fortieth birthday.

I was not a recovering ballet dancer or a gymnast or an acrobat. I was just recovering—mostly from the Sixties and Seventies. The Nineties were hard as well. I was a new mom, exhausted and carrying forty extra pounds. I had no idea what I was supposed to do with my life other than change diapers. I had just left a corporate job, which truthfully had become my entire existence, to raise a family, because one day a very little boy looked at me and asked me to please not go away anymore. When my friends at work heard I was firing the nanny, the gardener, the pool man, and my part-time maid/cook to do it all myself, they considered selling tickets to watch the show.

Compared to running a marketing division for a Fortune 100 company, my children's nursery was shockingly different. I had always been good at my job, but I kind of sucked at being at the beginning of my "mothering" journey. Above all, yoga made me a better mom. Now I know, every parent feels this way. We live each day analyzing how we spoke to our kids, scolded, or—God forbid—spanked, and failed to give a "life lesson" at a crucial moment that could have helped them get into Harvard. But back then I thought I was the only one.

Home alone while my husband traveled, I was coping with the demands of motherhood by sitting in the kitchen late at night eating Häagen Dazs ice cream with a vodka chaser. As if I didn't feel pathetic enough, we were living in Los Angeles where everyone is sort of gorgeous. I was the oldest mom with the youngest husband, and one of the few with her original equipment. And believe me, after nursing two healthy boys, my "girls" had seen better days. Every day I would wake up to the same old wash, rinse and repeat of my life and wonder, who the hell am I?

At forty, I had lost sight of my dreams. To find them again, I was going to have to awaken to who I was. Finding out who you are is everything in life.

Unfortunately, this journey involved making peace with the past, which kind of sucks. Right? I mean, if we all made peace with the past, there would be no need for therapists and every child of the Sixties and Seventies would no longer have anything to whine about. But running away from the past is like running away from you. It's just not an efficient route to happiness.

In the middle of feeling pathetic and sorry for myself, I was lucky to have discovered yoga. Like most people who come to the mat, I was looking for a way to feel better in my body. But instead, I found a path to feeling better in my heart. Transformation does not usually begin in the body, but the body is often what brings us to the mat. The body gets us there because we cannot touch our toes, or stand for a long time to make dinner, or carry a load of laundry up the stairs. Our mile is getting slower, our physical ability is on the decline, and in general, we are still young enough that we're not ready to give up. So we try yoga. Everyone says it works.

My journey into yoga began almost entirely by accident. I was looking for the Pilates room in my local gym and stumbled into a yoga class instead. (I've never been good with directions.) However in twelve years, I have not left. I practice yoga almost every day with the devotion of a Cenobite Monk. I went down the rabbit hole so far that today I teach yoga in two styles: Power and Hatha. I'm a writer and weekly columnist. I try to inspire others to find their inspiration on the mat and in their life.

You may notice that during this crazy journey of mine that I lost a lot of weight, I lost a certain "Eeyore" attitude, and I lost a kind of cynicism that permeated my outlook. But I want to be clear. *Finding More on the Mat* is not a story about weight loss or about loss of any kind in my life. My story is about finding more. Through yoga I've been able to transform my life from the "to do" list to the "to be" list. I remembered who I wanted to be. Yoga helps me to wake up and dream big. *Finding More* is my story on and off the mat. I hope it inspires others to stop wasting time and to live more fully every moment of their lives.

PART ONE

Growing Better

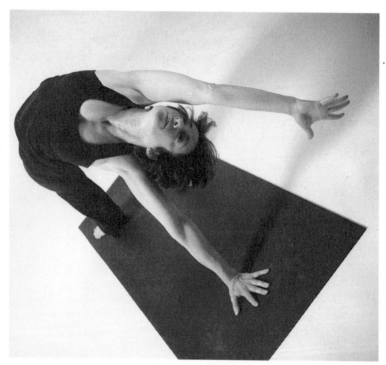

Pose: Wild Thing

Grace Is Everywhere

In the beginning, I did not know that I needed Grace.

After all, I had gone through the better part of my life without anything nearly looking like Grace. You should see me dance. Or sing. Oh My God. A goose suffering an epileptic attack would describe my attempts at being graceful. I would never be mistaken for a soul sister.

Then one day on my mat, struggling for the millionth time to touch my toes, I gave up. I kind of said, *"To hell with it."* And that's when it happened. The tension in my body released and I lowered down another six inches toward the floor. I got so excited I almost pulled a hamstring.

All the years I had been practicing yoga I thought what I needed to touch my toes and to get better in general was more effort. But in fact, I needed more Grace.

Grace is, in many ways, reflective of the attitude we bring to the mat. It is the difference between a yoga practice that leaves you radically transformed, and an exercise class. It's the difference between feeling full of hope and potential, and feeling like a schmuck. Our attitude creates the distinction between growing better on the mat, or feeling as if we're going to die every time we bend over.

When we take a yoga pose, it is not necessarily the shape of the thing that counts. Rather, it is a chance to create an offering of the highest intention in our hearts.

I learned on my mat that before I could get better, I would have to adjust my attitude. No matter how much I wanted the crazy poses, I would have to surrender my ego first. Before I could be a better parent, wife, friend and teacher, before I could love and serve better, I would have to live my yoga.

Living with ease is Grace. Living with forgiveness and acceptance is Grace. Taking the good with the bad is Grace. Saying "yes" first, rather than "no" is Grace. Trying new experiences with a light heart is Grace. Knowing that we are filled with forgiveness, *just because we were born,* is Grace.

Before you can radically transform the second half of your life, you'll have to go inside the first and forgive yourself for all of it. You will need equal parts of redemption and emancipation to find transformation, which is not easy. Today I am stronger and more vibrant than ever before. I hauled my tired old ass out of a steep depression to live a better life. I hope to make the second half of my life my best achievement yet.

The journey begins with Grace.

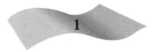

The Fearless Heart

I got me a fearless heart
Strong enough to get you through the scary part
It's been broken many times before
A fearless heart just comes back for more.
~ Steve Earle

"Yoga not easy."

That was a favorite saying of Sri K. Patabahi Jois, the founder of Ashtanga yoga.

Neither is love. That is what I've figured out.

At seventy-two years old, my mother, divorced for almost fifty years, decided to get married. Crazy! Right? But here I was listening to her giggling like a teenager on the phone. Usually when she calls me it's to say she's moving. Or she's going somewhere like Antarctica. So when she announced that she was getting married, I just had to ask:

"Are you knocked up?"

My Mom had been with her female partner for eighteen years; they had settled into a contented life. They are college professors and live three seasons a year near the universities where they work, and spend the summers traveling around the country. They were so comfortable that I never imagined they wanted to get married. For most of their lives it was illegal for women to marry, but apparently it wasn't illegal for them to dream about it.

Now a business trip to Canada made it possible. You may ask, after 18 years of living together, why bother? Because I certainly did. But despite the legal reasons why a couple may want to get married, none are more important than my mother jumping around her kitchen table and laughing like a teenager. I can't even remember the last time she walked without a cane.

That is how I came to be standing on a cliff in British Columbia looking out over the ocean on a truly magnificent day in the summer of 2010. I wasn't sure what to expect from a woman who has made shocking me an art form, but here she was, in a turquoise pantsuit sort of matching with her partner, who has now lived with her longer than I had growing up.

"Have you anything to say?" asked the Ceremony Officiate (that's Canadian for Justice of the Peace). I wanted to mention something about the matching turquoise outfits.

"Yes," said my Mom. "This time I want to be the husband." I was all ears. "I tried being the wife, and honestly, it wasn't a good deal. If I'm going to marry again, I want to be the husband."

And just like that, she became the "husband" in her new marriage. Oh, she had to rattle her cane and double-check the license, but if you look it up, it will say she is the "husband-wife" in this, her second and probably final marriage. Her partner has the exact same title, just to keep things on an even keel.

I don't care if you write it on a license or swear to God above, love is not easy, and rarely on an even keel. Call it what you want: wife, husband or husband-wife, or husband-husband, wife-wife. Love not easy. Love takes work.

Love is just like yoga:
You have to have a fearless heart.
And you have to be willing to fail
over and over again before you get it right.

Love Not Easy

My own track record at love is not so great.

My first husband left me after twenty months. I know, right? Twenty months. There are Hollywood marriages that last longer. It's hard to admit that Brittany Spears did better than I did at marriage. At one point I actually counted the days that I was joined in matrimonial bliss, but then decided that was not productive. These were twenty months, I might add, that I had spent moving around to accommodate his various jobs and step-parenting his child from an earlier marriage (which, I'm embarrassed to say, had lasted way longer than my paltry twenty months).

It seems that right after the honeymoon, while I was busy trying to figure out if I needed a Cuisinart food processor or a KitchenAid mixer to be a good wife, because we could not afford both (truthfully, we couldn't afford either), he was very busy with the wife of the former assistant city editor for the local Midwest newspaper.

Just like any other newly married bride, I was really worried that while the food processor could pulverize just about anything in seconds, the food mixer could make real bread dough! And I wasn't sure which one would be the better investment for my marriage. So I called my mother, which is what I do in times of crisis, and she asked me, what the hell was I doing in the kitchen? Right, I thought. She always put me back on track.

By then, twenty months into wedded bliss, my husband and I were living completely different lives. I was trying to become the kind of person who commutes an hour each way to work a ten-hour a day job, comes home to piles of laundry and dishes in the sink, makes dinner, and still wants sex with her husband. (You see the problem here, right?) I thought while I was gone twelve hours a day that he had been working late on the newspaper as a staff reporter to make a better life for us, or at least to help with the bills while he spent the mornings hanging around the house trying to write, what? A novel? A screenplay? A "roses are red" poem? Apparently not. It turned out that he was doing charitable work. He was spending his time helping the wife of the former assistant city editor, who had recently recovered memories that she may have been abused by her brother. She had taken many nights and a long weekend in an Indianapolis hotel to think about it some more, and my husband had been meeting her for some extra "thinking" time. I mean, who has an affair in Indianapolis? Not to be snooty, but if I have an affair I hope to God it's in Paris. Or Bora Bora.

This business of "recovered memories" happened in the Eighties, when it seemed everyone went to bed and woke up with a new discovery of earlier bad behavior. I personally think it might have been a delayed reaction to the Sixties and Seventies, depending on how many drugs you tried. I actually went to bed one night during this time and woke up to discover that my husband was not at home at 2 A.M., and thinking I might be recovering some kind of memory of being married, I drove around to find him. My search ended at a bar, where my husband was helping the former assistant city editor's wife recover his tongue from the back of her throat. And just like that, my marriage was pulverized in seconds, with or without the Cuisinart.

On moving day, when my soon to be ex-husband and his soon-to-be third wife were pulling out of the driveway of our tiny rented townhouse, I stood there in shocked disbelief. The whole break up had happened in the space of just one week. This was totally the wrong ending. It wasn't the version of my life where I had a white picket fence and 2.2 kids. I never saw it coming, but that's probably because I was busy with the blender decision.

The morning after I discovered the two of them kissing in a bar, when he told me she didn't mean anything to him, and that I had been imagining it, and that I was crazy, I was more than happy to believe him. Then that evening, when he said well perhaps I misunderstood, and that now he was in love with her, and that he never loved me, and he was moving with her in the morning to another Midwest newspaper, I laughed because I thought it was a joke. I have always had a problem with laughing at really inappropriate times. Funerals, final exams, visits to the gravely ill in the hospital will have me in stitches. But then he lectured me, with his face all puckered up in the serious way you look at a child who is just not getting it, that we both need to be nice to her because of her recovered memories.

Therefore, I was extremely polite to the former assistant city editor's wife as I watched her and my husband drive off in the car I paid for to their new home in the West, but I could not quite stifle a giggle. After they had completely disappeared and left me without a car, or a place to live, or even my job (long story), I had a really good laugh until I dissolved into long pathetic miserable sobs.

I mean, what was the point of working so hard at love if your husband is just going to leave you in the end for another woman?

"Look on the bright side," my best friend told me at the time. "He could have left you for another man." And we laughed some more until we cried.

You Will Fail Before You Get It Right

By the time I was thirty years old I had failed at love. I had failed at marriage. And now I had to return home to my parents, which if this has never happened to you, I want you to know totally sucks. But, unless I was in a Jane Austen novel, I was technically still young enough to try again.

My heart, however, was not so fearless. My heart was telling me that I should skip getting married all together. Due to economic circumstances (my ex taking me for everything I had, which was a car and an oriental rug I didn't really want), I returned home, tail between my legs. There is nothing quite like coming home in your thirties, brokenhearted, financially ruined, and dependent on your parents for a social life. My

Dad, who had advised me years earlier to go to business school and get an MBA, would introduce me as his oldest daughter who had screwed up her life with "this journalism business." Now I was the recently divorced daughter who could still go to business school, and by the way does anyone know of any single doctors?

But then something amazing happened. While I was divorced, stranded, and destitute, I started to make money! Not just enough to pay the rent on a tiny studio apartment, which as a writer is considered highly successful. *But real money.* Perhaps I needed to hit bottom so I could find a way to crawl out of the hole.

After my 20-month, 593-day marriage (I went ahead and counted the days, totally unproductive, but I had time on my hands), I took a job as a speechwriter for the CEO of a Fortune 100 company (needing money is perhaps the best motivator). Everything with the job was going well, so *of course* the CEO called me into his office one day to say he was going to be fired. Does this shit only happen to me? First my husband leaves me. Then *my boss, the CEO* is going to be fired. Before he left, he wanted to be sure I was going to be okay. Meanwhile, I was so *not okay.*

Since my marriage fell apart, I was staying with friends until I could scrape together enough money to move back home to New York; now my job was disappearing. I guess when the CEO is fired, they usually fire his speechwriter too. So he said that as of this minute, I was now being transferred to sales. "Even if you can't sell crap," he said, "it will take them a year to find you."

That sounded good to me. Give me a year to hide and feel sorry for myself. I got a raise (because apparently even brand new sales trainees who know nothing make more than writers who have an Ivy League degree) and went through basic sales training.

And then, astonishingly, I was good at it! Who could have guessed that I would thrive at sales? It turned out, I was able to speak on the phone for hours on the subject of things I knew nothing about, because talking about nothing is something I can do very well.

From the Midwest I was sent to New York to cover the financial services industry. So although the job was a ticket for me to go home again, it turned out I was unbelievably successful. Dad is still in shock. For the first time in my adult life, I could eat in a restaurant that had tablecloths! I could afford an apartment! I could even take a taxi, although truthfully I'm more of a walker unless it's late at night.

The other result of being independent is that for the first time, I did not need a man. I would have liked a horse, as I rode most weekends and sometimes after work, but a man would have just gotten in the way in those days.

When you don't need something, that's when you get it.

It happens in yoga all the time. You want a pose, and then just when you give up on the idea of ever getting your foot behind your head, pop—there it goes. Yoga teaches us that desire can help achieve your dreams, but too much also takes you off track. When you want something, but can also be content to live without it, that's when the Universe may choose to make good on your wish.

Therefore, when I really did not want a man on any kind of permanent basis, the Universe made good on a wish I didn't make. I met Mike on a blind date on a Friday night. By Sunday afternoon, we seriously needed food. (You will have to read between the lines, because there is a very good chance my kids will read this book, even though I haven't actually seen them read any book since the videogame was invented.) Honestly, I didn't know that what I wanted was a Montana man with an MBA. So I told him I didn't think this would go anywhere because there's nothing like an out-of-town boyfriend to take you away from what you wanted most: a decent paycheck!

Mike, however, has that Western "can-do" spirit. As far as he's concerned, there isn't a mountain that can't be climbed and a horse that can't be broken. He once caught a fish with his bare hands. (I saw it, although truthfully, the fish might have been a little under the weather.) So either it was my raving intellect or all the beer we drank that weekend, but he took me as a challenge and we were married six months later.

Marriage Not Easy

After two marriages you would think I would know something more about love and life, and even about myself, but sadly, it's not so. It took yoga to set me straight.

By the time I found yoga, I was forty years old, and *so completely* lost that I was on the school parent organization volunteering to bake cookies. I mean, what the hell?

Remember, I don't know how to use the food processor thing because my mother told me to get out of the kitchen.

Furthermore, if you knew me, you would realize I should not be around children for extended periods of time, especially other people's children, and not just because of my New York City fondness for the "F" word. I have this little problem with patience, although it seems to get better with vodka. However, I am way more tolerant with children than I am with most of the parents who were debating for two hours whether the children should spend Valentine's Day making gifts for a Native American reservation or for the Children's Hospital. *"Are you freaking kidding me?"* I asked the PTO [Parent Teacher Organization], and for some reason all eyes were suddenly on *moi!* "We are talking about six year olds! Give them a cookie and call it a day."

I was still impersonating Mother Teresa at school and Martha Stewart at home when I woke up and realized I was not happy. By now, in my second marriage, I had both the Cuisinart and the KitchenAid and was determined to learn how to use them to do these incredibly useful things, like bake bread, which takes something like fifty-five hours when you can go to the store and buy some in fifteen minutes.

Husband: "Let's have sex."

Me: "Would love to, but I need to punch down the bread in ten minutes."

Do we really wonder why Martha Stewart is divorced?

By the time I came to yoga, I had absolutely no idea who I was anymore. I loved my husband, I loved my children, but I can't say that I loved myself. Even my mother was worried that I was trying to bake cookies. So I got out of the kitchen,

I stopped volunteering at school (strange, but no one called to say they missed me), and I got on my mat.

Yoga Is a Window Inside

From almost the first class I took, I devoted myself completely to this new weird and wonderful passion. Yoga consumed my every waking moment, except of course when I had to make breakfast, lunch, dinner, do the laundry, drive carpool, help with homework and pick up after the dogs. But even during this new stage of my life, I started to feel like me again, whoever that was. When I became a mother I had the opportunity to do better. I may not be the best mother (clearly), but I was thinking that with a little effort, I could create a perfect caring, enlightened little person on the planet, and the world would be a better place. My plan was going great until the kids turned two and learned the word "no." Then it all went to shit.

**If yoga not easy, and love not easy,
then being a good mother—nearly impossible.**

Creating perfect little humans was not working out for me, so I was going to have to find another way to spend my time. I often wonder if I had not found yoga, whether I would have inflicted all my hopes and desires on my kids, and what a terrible burden that would have been. Luckily, without *my* ambitions, they are free to find their own.

And so I hit the mat in earnest. In the beginning, it was sixty minutes out of the house to ease my aching back. Then

I started to connect with something bigger. This was my first hit of Grace.

Outside the yoga room, it was crazy and hysterical, a whirlwind of diapers and snacks and activities and laundry and work and, and, and.... But on the mat, it was quiet. This time was for me. Each pose became an expression of the love and faith in my heart, even if I couldn't yet express my new optimism off the mat. Each pose was an opportunity to be so much better than I thought I could be on my own. If I offered a little prayer to God, or dedicated a pose to someone I love, or honored my teacher with my best effort, it became enormous with potential. I am not just a pretzel, but I'm a person *in love with her potential,* and crazy enough to see how far she can go. Who am I? What can I achieve? Is there a limit, or am I limitless? This is a glimpse of not just the greater human I can be, but of the Divine in me. How else can we explain what we are able to do on the mat?

With yoga, I am able to see that I am not just Michelle, the laundress, the cook, the driver, sleeping like a homeless person in the back seat of the car during soccer practice. I am MICHELLE, a child of GOD, who can do ANYTHING, and she CHOOSES to sleep in the car at this moment with her feet hanging out the window. It is a subtle difference, but one is a dead-end to hopelessness, and one is to be absolutely present, totally divine and with a purpose.

Discover the Divine Within

What is Grace? And how do we get it? Beyond touching my toes, or healing my back, that was the primary challenge of my early yoga practice. The more I heard yoga teachers talking about Grace, the more I knew I wanted some. So I kept asking, *who do I have to kill around here to get some motherfucking Grace?*

Apparently, all you need to do to find Grace is to shut up, which explains why I had such a hard time finding it. All the talk, the noise, the "busy-ness," the running around, the electronic intrusions in our lives are giant distractions from the real issue at hand: finding peace. But that is exactly what we need more of in our lives: more contentment with the moment; more acceptance of what is; more recognition for where you are, wherever that is. That is all Grace.

It helps to be quiet and listen to find Grace. So before each yoga practice, in fact before each pose, I take a moment to tune in. I use breath to listen up and see how I feel and where I am. I practice to find Grace. Once I connected with Grace on the mat, I was able to see it in my life.

When I feel Grace is with me, it is as if the Universe enters my soul and fills me up with promise. I am exploding with potential. I thought I had so much potential as a kid. We all did. I could do anything, and often did. I had several careers, moved around and traveled the world. I've ridden racehorses (true), sailed 50-foot yachts (also true), and skied the Rocky Mountains (so true, I can race you to the bottom). And then I traded everything for a life in the suburbs. I felt a little lost.

Then one day I got on my mat and I felt peace, and I felt purpose, and I felt a little bit of a challenge. From the beginning I realized, *here* is something that would take a lifetime of devotion to learn. I was so ready. Crazy enough, this clarity brought focus to my life off the mat as well. I had a renewed energy for my family in a way I didn't think possible.

**Yoga is my path for endless remembrance
of who I am and what I want in life.**

Just as my mother may have dreamed of getting married again, I too had dreams. I wanted more out of life, for myself and for my family. A fearless heart never gives up.

A Lesson From the Mat

Be Willing To Fail

"Love is like yoga: You have to be prepared to do it over and over again," said my teacher, Chris Muchow. "And when you fail, you have to be strong enough to try again."

To practice yoga is to be willing to fail. With any pose that you struggle with over and over, the pose is never the point; it is what it reveals about the self that keeps you coming back.

I once took a workshop with a teacher who did not do her first Handstand, *Adho Mukha Vrksasana*, until she was in her fifties. She was giving a workshop on Handstands, and demonstrating a press-up variation that involves a tremendous amount of core strength, perseverance and balance. Although she floated up, rather effortlessly, she confessed that it took her something like 6,337 times to get it. How did she know? She kept a journal and counted the attempts.

Press-Up Handstand is also my Mount Everest. I work at this pose several times a week, often quite unsuccessfully. There are ten-year-old gymnasts and twenty-year-old yoga teachers who can press out a Handstand every five minutes. Face it, the pose itself is not that special, unless it took you 6,337 times to get there. I am willing to try, because I'm also willing to fail. Getting up and trying again is the first step to success on the mat.

The great thing about failing, even failing over and over again, is if you do it enough you might just learn something. If you take the time to consider what holds you back in a pose, and what you allow to hold you back, you will unlock the secret to finding your power.

A Lesson From the Mat

Awaken to Who You Are

When I practice, it's to remember my fearless heart. Every time I practice, I cultivate a steadfast remembrance of who I was, who I am, and who I have yet to be. It is easy to lose perspective in all the noise of your life.

If there is joy in getting older (because there certainly is little delight in looking in the mirror), it is this: I finally know who I am. I know my strengths, and weaknesses. I know when to get help and when I can offer help. This is liberating.

Somewhere along the line, in the kitchen, the laundry room, the boardroom, the pre-school classroom, "Michelle" had gotten a little lost. It is probably true for all of us. But on my mat, I found "me" again. When it was challenging, I found willpower. To find balance, I connected with inner strength. When I was afraid, I practiced calm. And in meditation, I found answers.

Yoga has taught me that I am not good at all things, and that's okay. I am better at the strength poses, and need help with flexibility. I am strong in inversions, and need to work on backbends. My hips are open, but my hamstrings are tight. One person is never good at all things, but knowing where you need help is the beginning to growing better on your mat.

A Lesson From the Mat

Remember Why You Came

At first, we practice yoga because it makes us feel better in our bodies. Then, it transforms us as we find a spiritual path to Grace.

Knowing ourselves, recognizing our gifts and being able to love more clearly becomes its own reward. Our lives are enhanced, and we in turn, enhance those around us. Once I discovered this in yoga, it was hard to imagine my life without it.

Ultimately, this is Grace. It is recognizing the divine qualities in each of us. It is abundance, and forgiveness, and love. It is everything, and exists solely in nothing. If you can tap into Grace, then you can tap into that quality of infinite possibility for yourself.

While I came to my mat for all sorts of reasons, I stayed for mainly one: I thought I might at long last live up to my potential. When we get a little "hit" of the Universe and just how beautiful it is to be part of it, we get a vision of ourselves at our best. When I practice, I always bear in mind: *Give to the highest first.* I give to the love of my family. I offer to my children and their ability to grow into their potential. I give to my loved ones everywhere. I give to my community, which in turn, gives so much to me. But most of all, I give to the Divine. The chance to fill up with Grace, to be lifted up with something divine, is a chance to wake up to our fullest potential.

We may come to our mats because something in our life is broken. We stay, because yoga wakes us up to more.

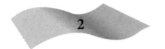

Cit Happens

You can't be brave
if you've only had wonderful things happen to you.
~ Mary Tyler Moore

I would not say it was love at first sight when I saw my son. It was more like panic.

Most new mothers will tell you about how beautiful their babies are (me, too), and how perfect they are (me, too). My baby was also brilliant, I could tell from his eyes. (They were mine!) He was serene (I learned later that was from the delivery drugs), and surely the most ideal human being ever. And in the moment of beholding such a tiny fragile child, I knew I was going to screw this up. I had no idea how I was going to keep him out of harm's way. So instead of delighting in the moment, I pulled the covers over my head and disappeared into a three-day morphine bender courtesy of Los Angeles' Cedars Sinai Hospital. (When the delivery involves a close encounter with an electric saw to break apart your pelvis to get the baby out, you get as much morphine as you want, along with a bill for $100,000.)

Somehow, Sam survived and continued to thrive despite my parenting, which began with morphine-tainted breast milk. Not many mothers can say they've fed their babies

Class A felony drugs right from the get-go. I followed that up with allowing him to eat the school lunches. (Now that he's a teenager, he can proudly tell you the differences between a Big Mac and an In-N-Out Double Double.)

I live in the suburbs where mothers compete to see who made their young children the purest organic lunches, who went to school to watch them eat their vegetables, who played the most politically correct gender neutral games at recess (which usually included their own children being picked for captains). Seriously, *I can't make this stuff up.* I have friends who still eat with their children in middle school. Can you imagine being fourteen years old and having lunch every day with your mommy?

Apparently, there are a lot of women who have nothing to do in my part of town. And once they realized I put my children on the bus and let them eat the school lunch, I was off the list for mother's night out.

By the time my second child was born, I was better off. I realized the hopelessness of keeping him 100% organic, so I asked the delivery room doctors for the morphine right away. Apparently, when it is a textbook delivery with no complicating factors, they don't give you the drugs. That is when I panicked, again. I did not anticipate being completely sober and bringing yet another vulnerable baby into the world.

This is the nature of life. There is the joy of looking into your infant's eyes—that's *ananda*, Sanskrit for bliss. Then there is *cit*, consciousness or truth (and yes, it's pronounced like chit to make sure you understand what it's really like)—reality. *Cit* is the realization that you will probably screw this up. You must try to keep this little person safe and healthy.

You are responsible for getting him to maturity, and possibly finding some way to pay for the ridiculous cost of a college education. But once the hospital cut me off the morphine, the *cit* was overwhelming. I had to turn to alcohol and prescription drugs to be a good mother. That was before I found yoga.

If you are alive, then you are aware of *cit*. I can do my best to protect my children, but really, I know it's useless. I can feed them organic foods, buy them down coats, and teach them about stranger danger. But in the end, what can we really control? They still forget their homework, or fail their exams, or break an arm, and then break it again. They play gallantly at sports, then tear an ACL [anterior cruciate ligament] and spend a year on the bench. They leave their coats at home on the coldest days, and run across the street without looking both ways. They compete and win, and they compete and fail. Sometimes they bounce back, sometimes they don't. Although my parents tried to protect me and do what they thought was best, still *cit* happens. It is never anybody's fault. It is life. We persevere because the alternative isn't so great either.

Embrace Your Stain to Have It All

One day I was sitting on my mat obsessed about what was holding me back in my practice. That is usually how I practice yoga, obsessed with all my negatives and faults and shortcomings.

I was having trouble with backbends. Not just one pose, the whole stinking posse of poses was eluding me. I could not "melt the heart." To melt the heart, you must pull the shoulder blades onto your back, and at the same time move the chest forward so the upper back becomes supple. For stiff people, this action is like softening concrete; you cannot muscle your way into the pose. You have to "melt." You have to "dissolve." You have to "liquefy." It had to be "easy." *Right? What the hell?* This was ridiculous.

My shoulders were tight and rounded from fifty years of self-consciousness. I had the spinal curvature of an eighty year old. I already had the hump that took my grandmother from a lanky 5'5" to a diminutive 4'6" in her last few years.

I knew as a yogi, I should be tirelessly working to save the world, but at that moment, I was trying to save myself. And it was doubtful.

So I was sitting on my mat feeling pathetic when my teacher told a story about the Goddess Lakshmi, who once upon a time also had a very bad day. In Hinduism, Lakshmi is the Goddess of abundance, wealth and beauty; basically she is the Heidi Klum of the ancient world. She had it all.

One day Lakshmi was invited to a wedding and she picked out a beautiful white dress. But as she put it on, she began her menstrual cycle and accidentally got a stain on it. Horrified, she went into hiding and withdrew from the world. But without her abundance and radiance shining on the earth, the sun faded, the crops withered, and the world began to die.

It fell to the God Shiva to save the earth. He was angry that while Lakshmi was worried about her little dress, the world was withering away. Shiva told her, "You have got to end this suffering; it's not all about you and your silly little dress." (I'm improvising here because although I am old, I am not *that* old to have been there 2,000 years ago.) This was about the world's abundance.

So Lakshmi decided if she could not get the stain out of her dress, if it was now part of the fabric, then she would *embrace it and make it beautiful.* She dyed her dress a brilliant red. Her beauty was not only restored, she actually became breathtaking.

We are not made less by our little imperfections, we are made more. And if we can use the blemishes in our life to make ourselves more brilliant, then we *become* Lakshmi.

I sat on my mat, stunned.

If the world's most beautiful and wealthy Goddess could embrace her stain, then I guess so could the rest of us mere mortals.

For so long I thought I was the only one with something to hide! I suddenly realized that everyone has a stain. Everyone has something they'd rather not talk about. This must be a part of the human condition.

In an instant, I realized that part of growing up and growing better, would be to accept who I was, imperfections and all. Acceptance and forgiveness were going to be the way. This is very hard for Type A's. We expect a lot, perfection in fact. I would much rather ignore any issues and push on in life than deal with so much unpleasantness! After all, I have successfully ignored the hump on my back for years by simply not looking behind me in the mirror.

Yet I realized, if I was going to make progress on my mat, I would have to peel away my layers of protection and unearth the problem. I very much wanted to do backbends and inversions, but my heart would not melt. Partly it was the hump, and partly it was because my right arm simply did not work as well as my left. I could not pull the shoulder into my body for support. It was stuck. And worse, now that I was in my fifties, the imbalance from my shoulders was creating a pain down the right side of my back. I was living in real physical pain and experiencing a blockage on my mat from something that I suspect may have started in my head.

I knew I was bigger than this. Like Lakshmi, I could figure this out and fix it. And so I did. It was time to stop hiding my *cit*, dye my dress and wear it to the party.

The Spirit Survives All

The hump in my back and the problem with my arm did not happen overnight. As in my case, the seeds for these things were usually planted long before they materialized.

My father was born to a modest family and became a successful uptown Park Avenue veterinarian in New York City. My mother was born to a wealthy family and wanted to be a free spirit in the downtown scene emerging on Christopher Street in Greenwich Village. Why they divorced was easy to understand; why they ever got married was more confusing. My father was stable and upright. My mother was experimenting. She was in her twenties, single, and (there's no other way to describe it), a joyful, wild woman. She was a writer, a photographer and a would-be opera singer. She joined various theater companies, travelled across the country—twice—sold everything to live on a boat, then sold the boat to live on land again, all the while toting a child.

I was becoming adept at moving between these two worlds. Uptown on Park Avenue, I could curtsey for the adults and dress for dinner. Downtown, in Greenwich Village, or on the boat, or in Long Island, I ate my TV dinners during poetry readings.

Although having a double life gave me more exposure to the world, it also had its downside. By the time I was twelve, my mother and I had lived in a dozen places—including the boat. I would miss school, a lot of school, probably at least two years of school, as Mom would frequently take me out to go on her adventures. My "Auntie Mame" Mom would say that life teaches us more than any room with four walls, however school officials thought otherwise. By the time I was in sixth grade, my father had had enough. My gypsy lifestyle was going to end.

The compromise as to who would be a better parent was to send me away. *Go figure.* Reluctantly, my mother packed me up and drove me to a boarding school in upstate New York for the seventh grade. This would provide me with stability, respectability and a good education, so we all thought.

I was young for my grade, only twelve years old, and having spent a mostly solitary childhood with my mother, I was still playing with my Barbies and my magic oven in middle school. After my mother, the biggest influence in my life was my grandmother, Sarah, a woman who matched my bags and shoes from an early age. At twelve, I thought shopping with my grandmother on Fifth Avenue was about the greatest pleasure a girl could have.

September arrived bringing in the new school year, so I packed my dresses and matching shoes in a large trunk. (Mom said we could use it to travel on a ship someday, and that was a dream I clung to for many lonely nights at school.) With hair in a neat ponytail and barrettes that matched my blouse, I got into Mom's candy apple red convertible and drove 600 miles to a school that was literally, a pig farm. *I cannot make this stuff up.*

You may ask, how did a girl with matching shoes, bags and barrettes get to a pig farm? That's a very good question. Truly, there were more than just pigs on the farm. There were also horses, cows, chickens, mice and cats, but once you are greeted by the smell of a dozen pigs, you will never forget it.

In the early 1970s, during the anti-war make-love fervor that gripped much of the country, it was briefly considered the thing to do to send the wealthy offspring of Manhattan liberals to live in progressive boarding schools that were structured like communes. Everyone worked. In the mornings we had barn chores and so I tottered up the hill at dawn in my ridiculous shoes with the prim heels to slaughter the pigs and wring the chickens' necks. Imagine a girl from Park Avenue or even Greenwich Village holding a dead chicken? Of course, there were lots of children attending, not just the urban expats from New York City, but also a few local children, a few scholarship children, and as it turned out, a budding psychopath.

Although I tried, I could not eat the food I had actually fed in the morning. I looked at the bacon on the dining table and threw up. By the early afternoon I was starving, so I would go begging the kitchen staff for something to eat. On occasion, I would sneak into the dorm parents' private residences and raid their refrigerator. I guess technically this was stealing, but I was desperate for food. Apparently, the rules were that the students were only allowed to eat the animals they slaughtered and the organic food they planted, but the staff could stock their private refrigerators with snacks of all kinds.

In retrospect, I learned a lot about the true nature of Communism. On the surface, everyone pretended that we shoveled the shit together, but in private, those with power kept the Twinkies for themselves.

Whenever I got in trouble, it involved food. I was caught stealing it, hiding it, smuggling it, and worst of all, not eating it at the table. I hid on the slaughterhouse days, and then was punished by being sent to my room without dinner. I begged my mother to send me food, and then her packages would be confiscated. She'd get the call from the headmaster that once again her daughter was caught with illegal, non-organic food.

"Let me get this straight," she told the headmaster on the phone while I sat in detention. "My daughter is in trouble because she's hungry? What the hell is wrong with you people?"

I love my mother.

From then on I was allowed to get an afternoon snack if I was hungry. Even though I had won the war with the school's food police, I was still miserable. I tried to make it better by getting some boots for barn chores so I would not have to muck the stalls in my patent leather Mary Janes. (When I asked Mom to buy me some kind of barn boot, she replied, "If Bloomingdales doesn't have these things, you are out of luck, because there's no way in hell I'm going to New Jersey." New Jersey was the wild, wild West where they would have barn boots.) But as to the true depth of my misery, I felt I could not tell anyone. I knew my unhappiness would cause my parents, especially my mother and grandmother, more heartache. I knew I would have to tough it out. I was going to have to put on a stiff upper lip and survive the year.

And then it got worse, because *of course* it does.

It started at the back door of the kitchen one afternoon while I was waiting for my food handout. While my mother and I expected that perhaps I might have a piece of toast or a peanut butter sandwich, I was usually given a carrot or a piece of cooked potato. If you averaged the cost of tuition by the food, that potato was worth about a hundred bucks.

I am standing by the kitchen door for my bite of potato when the leader of a pack of boys came prowling around the corner. This was not Peter Pan. This was a pimply-faced sixteen year old with greasy black hair, a red headband and dirty Levis. He must have been left back in his grade three times to be sixteen in middle school. And he had three more lost boys in tow.

"What have we got here?" he asked.

I would rather not tell the rest of the story, except that I've spent a lot of time pretending it didn't happen, and frankly, I'm tired of hiding the truth. All rapes are different, but they leave their victims the same: with a deep sense of loss and shame. For me, I lost my inner light for a while. There was an innocence and fearlessness in my heart that was taken from me. There was a clear before and after in my life. Most of all, I lost my trust in the world. The girl who waited with shoulders thrown back and head held high for the slice of cold potato because she had won the war with the school officials, was no longer. From that day forward, I walked hunched over keeping myself protected inside. The lesson I learned was that if you walk too proud, you might get hurt.

However, my story has a happy ending. So I need to tell it.

I remember the walk down the hall as the leader grabbed my right arm and twisted it tightly behind my back. The younger boys trotted behind us as he half-pushed, half-carried me to the boys' bathroom. Although I was afraid, I tried to keep my game face. Initially I thought he might want my potato! I told myself, this will be okay; it's only food. Then I told myself, I'm still okay; it's only my shoulder that feels broken. I'm still okay, my arm is numb but I can feel my fingers. I'm still okay; my heart is beating. And so on.

Once in the bathroom he threw me onto the floor and pulled my jeans down around my ankles. It took him several tries to get the job done. He kept my arm bent behind my back and the pain from my shoulder kept me from feeling anything else. Then the pain went away.

In fact, everything seemed to go away. My head was pushed up against the base of the toilet and I remember staring at the urine dried in yellow streaks along the base and thinking, *does anyone clean this bathroom?* But I didn't feel a thing. I had left my body. The girl on that bathroom floor was someone else. My spirit had risen. I could see what he was doing, I could hear what he was saying, but the whole thing was happening outside me.

"Let's see if this will fit," he said, poking me with his fingers, and then something else, I wasn't sure. Perhaps he used a broom. I can't say for sure. Somehow he found a way to do what he came to do. I was twelve years old, a virgin, and weighed less than 100-pounds. I was no match for him and so sexually inexperienced that I wasn't even sure of what was happening. And when it was over, I was a mess. Talk about a stain. My legs were covered in blood. My pants, which were still caught around my ankles, were soaked. There was so much blood I thought I might be dying. I hadn't yet had a period, and this was the first sight of female blood I'd ever seen.

Afterward, he stood at the sink and washed his hands. He fixed his bandana in the mirror and smoothed his greasy hair. Then he turned to his crew who were waiting at the door and said, "Your turn."

Grace Is Everywhere

Although this was the worst moment of my young life, I realized in that instant that just as I had been telling myself on that long trip down the hallway, *I was okay*. For whatever else would happen that day, and for the rest of my life, I knew this: I had survived. I thought that perhaps God was with me and allowed me to live. At that moment I did not know if I could be pregnant, or if my arm was seriously injured, or even if my insides were okay. But I knew this for sure:

We are bigger than the stuff that happens to us.

The spirit is not easily destroyed. I was okay, and I was going to be okay, no matter what else happened in this room, or for that matter, the rest of my life. I believed in God, and I believed that He might have spared me because I still had things to do in this world.

So as Mr. Red Bandana turned to the boys and said, "Your turn," I felt some twinge of hope. It's ridiculous, but this was perhaps my first hit of Grace. It was possibly the worst time of my life, but in the time it took him to turn around, I thought, *maybe this will be "my turn" to live.* And I promised myself I would seek revenge by living the rest of my life extremely well. It was my *cit-ananda* moment.

But at first, I did nothing. Survival was at the top of my list. I thought my arm might be broken because I could not move it. I was so bloody that I didn't know if this was a virginity thing or if I was hemorrhaging. So I decided to play dead, not a big stretch, but one of the best decisions of my life. I thought to myself, if I die, then it changes everything. We go from "boys being boys," (which was what the school called it when it was discovered that he'd done the same thing to a half dozen girls), to "boys being psychopaths" who have sex with dead underage girls. Right? I lay there while the other boys took a good, long look.

Take a good look you little sons of bitches, I thought to myself. *That's right; take a good look, because I hope this picture stays with you for the rest of your lives. Here, let me spread my legs a little wider so you can see exactly what was done to me.*

Then they ran.

And like a white dove the magician releases into the air, I was free. My heart fluttered and soared. My body was collapsed on the bathroom floor, but my spirit was high. Somehow I had just stopped this train from being an express. I had stopped just short of becoming the girl who did the track team. I was alive, and generally, okay.

Don't let me give the impression that everyone should experience a sexual trauma to know redemption. There are easier ways. It's taken me years of therapy to come to terms with it. When I did accept it, I didn't want to discuss it because it was never the thing that defined me. I have accomplished so much with my life, but everything else becomes secondary when you say the word "rape." Believe me, saying you were raped is a conversation stopper.

In all honesty, I do have a few regrets. The worst part is that I spent some time cleaning up the bathroom. This is so me. When I am stressed you will find me cleaning the house. What was I thinking? I should have been screaming and running down the hall Carrie style throwing blood on all the teenage jerks in the school. But instead, I was wiping the floor with paper towels.

Secondly, I regret not telling my parents what happened. I knew my mother would fall apart. She never wanted to me to go away in the first place and now she would worry terribly if I had to stay. I just called and said I needed to come home and see a doctor. I wasn't close enough to my father to talk about it.

Worse yet, by not saying what had really happened, I spent a lot of time listening to lectures from various adults about what they assumed happened. The school faculty and various therapists told me how important it was to wait to have sex until you meet the right one. *(Gosh, adults are soooo smart!)* I wanted the whole thing to disappear and to get back to my exciting life of mucking out the barns and eating cold potatoes. If I felt any shame, it was because I was not strong enough to have fought him off in the first place.

I don't regret my years of hiding, of being shy, of holding myself in and back from experiencing more of life. I don't regret not telling people I was raped. I needed time to figure it out. I didn't want to be a victim. I didn't feel like a victim.

For a while I felt like an idiot—because I shouldn't have been in that place, at that time. But a victim? Never. In the opera the victim ends up dying. Even at twelve I knew I survived something. I think the experience was the beginning of what made me who I am today.

Everything Heals with Love

A lifetime later, I was sitting on my mat in yoga class listening to the story of Lakshmi and suddenly I got it. I understood why I couldn't melt my heart in practice. Maybe there was something to this yoga stuff? Maybe I had trouble being vulnerable? Maybe I was afraid to be open and soft because if I showed that I am weak then my arm will be pulled behind my back and I will be dragged down the hall. And of course, for forty years I didn't walk upright because there was always the nagging thought, that if I stand up straight and walk with confidence, I could be "asking for it."

A light went on.

I realized that if I was to move forward, and to live out my promise to *live an extraordinarily good life*, I was going to have to find my spirit again. But not only would I have to find the swing in my hips, I would also need to be vulnerable, to get my trust on. Trying to control everything and protect myself so I wouldn't be hurt again honestly hadn't gone so well for me.

I was going to have to find some faith that the Universe, or God, or the Tooth Fairy would be there for me. *Oy Vay.*

While my spirit barely survived the attack, my right arm was truly a mess. My shoulder was separated on that bathroom floor, and as a result of resolutely ignoring it for decades, it never healed correctly.

This arm had been the source of so much frustration for me in my yoga practice. It resisted the rotation in Half Pigeon, *Eka Pada Raja Kapotasana*. It would not bend for Reverse Namaskar, *Paschima Namaskarasana*. I could not bind this arm behind me for Cow Face, *Gomukhasana*. And worst of all, in my inversions I could not pull this arm into my shoulder socket as deeply as my left, and so when I am upside down, I look like the leaning tower of Pisa. Even in Upward Facing Wheel, *Urdhva Dhanurasana*, the pain in my right shoulder was a showstopper. It could take my breath away, so it was a wonder why it took me so long to hear it. But really, I am a terrible listener; everyone says so.

When the light went on, I realized I had not dealt with this part of my past but buried it instead. Not only had I put every vestige of this incident behind me with a vengeance, I had actually forgotten about my arm! As I sat in yoga class listening to how important it is to accept our flaws, to practice with reverence for the whole picture, to love ourselves wholly and absolutely, it came to me. I realized, *oh my God, my shoulder was damaged by this lunatic!* I had never put two and two together. Why won't my arm do this? Because it was broken and now it needs to heal.

Later that morning, when it was time for inversions, my teacher picked Forearm Stand, *Pincha Mayurasana* for the practice. The exercise was to come up next to a wall and place your tail onto the hard surface. As you push backwards against the foundation, the heart melts forward. This is a deep heart opener. As I was working into my lopsided left-leaning posture, my teacher approached me. With sensitivity he placed his hand on the back of my right shoulder blade. "You need to bring this arm closer to your heart," he said.

For the first time in years, I started to cry. He probably thought my tears were about my tendencies to stray toward perfection. But no. I was upset at the years I wasted when I wouldn't pull my arm into my heart. I was upset at how much time I spent in denial, trying to be strong. I was upset that I couldn't remember if I had ever truly grieved for what had happened. I was upset that I had never really offered forgiveness to that part of myself. My arm was now the weakest part of my practice. I was damaged, but worse, I wouldn't forgive myself for being weak, and so I couldn't pull that part of myself into my heart.

That was it. I decided it was time to let this stuff go. Then, even if it killed me, I was going to pull that arm in and nurture it to health. I forgave myself for any part I had in being weak on that bathroom floor, and for possibly even liking that boy a little tiny bit before he did what he did.

Now, rather than feeling frustration, I feel love for my right arm. It is the best and worst of me. It symbolizes everything that I have survived, everything I am, and hope to still become. My once broken shoulder is my *cit-ananda*. Before I practice, I bring my right arm behind my back stretching it up in an act of deep remembrance and respect. Before inversions, I plug it in to the shoulder socket a little tighter, keeping it close to my heart. I get regular massage from a woman I love and trust. Whenever she breaks up the old scar tissue in that shoulder she says, "What the hell is in here?"

"Trust me, you don't want to know!" I answer.

After being hopelessly blocked for almost forty years, my arm is slowly coming around. Loving this arm, caring for it, accepting it as I do my total self, has provided me more freedom and joy than any amount of therapy.

Cit is consciousness or truth. It is facing up to what you may not want to know, particularly about yourself. But, it's also the part of life that if we survive it, we grow better. *Cit* is hard to avoid, although certain meds help. But in the end, you may not want to avoid the *cit*, because with radical understanding, comes radical freedom and growth.

Ananda is bliss. It is the deliciousness in life. The best moments of bliss usually come with some effort and are more rewarding than the pleasures that come easily to us.

These days I've come to a place where I welcome the *cit* as the *ananda*. I have come to a place where seeing clearly and accurately, without any illusions, has become my biggest pleasure. I am done with hiding. The change in my attitude has allowed me to be more serene in the good times, and more accepting of the bad times, and therefore life becomes *cit-ananda* more of the time. Life becomes a blissful acceptance of reality, a true *cit-ananda*.

Yoga Shines the Light

Because I wanted a deeper backbend, yoga helped me understand my story. My practice has shined a light into my soul. I feel like my own person again. I can be the outrageous, funny and radiant woman I was always meant to be. I don't have to be afraid that by standing tall, I'll be singled out and hurt again. I am so much smarter and more aware; it simply won't happen, or at least it won't happen that way again.

**The truth of the matter is,
if you live long enough, you will be hurt.**

We are all a little damaged. When I look at my precious children, I cannot bear the thought of them suffering. I try to keep them safe, as my parents tried but were unable in the end. When my boys are unfairly treated by life, I try to reign in my fears. I know every moment of pain is a chance for them to understand and grow stronger. It may be their *cit-ananda* moment and it's impossible, and perhaps even wrong, to take that away.

Life's bumps and bruises leave these little dents on our hearts and bodies, but it is our right to feel better. We can learn to use these experiences to polish our hearts to greater brilliance. We can use our body awareness to gain greater spirituality. My practice thrives, even though my heart does not melt as much as

I'd like, and my shoulder is a little rough in the rotation. That I can learn to thrive with my imperfections is yoga. Pain may be physical, or it may be emotional, the body doesn't differentiate. The work for the student is to understand, to listen and to accept. Then the work of growing better has begun. That is finding *cit-ananda* in life.

A Lesson From the Mat

How To Melt a Broken Heart

Melting the heart or bringing the shoulder blades onto the back while the upper chest softens and moves forward, is the key to backbends and many inversions.

- Cat/Cow stretch in tabletop position. With very strong arms, softly press your chest toward the ground. Then reverse the motion to stretch through the rhomboids.
- Stand at the wall, press your hands into the wall and with strong arms melt your heart forward.
- Lie on the floor, belly up, and place a yoga brick beneath your shoulder blades. Allow the heart to rise upward as you move the shoulders downward.
- Forearm stand, *Pincha Mayurasana*, at the wall (can also be done in Headstand, *Sirsasana*, and Handstand, *Adho Mukha Vrksasana)*. Bring the tailbone to the wall. Firmly lift the tailbone to the sky. At the same time, press your heart forward and your armpits back.

Go slow. Have patience and you will see improvement. The work is to understand, not necessarily to succeed right away. From understanding comes freedom.

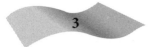

Stupid Human Tricks

Between the great things we cannot do,
and the small things we will not do,
the danger is that we shall do nothing.
~ Adolphe Monod

Yoga is humbling. The more you practice, the less you feel you know.

When I first came to the mat, I decided pretty quickly I was an "advanced" student. I came to this conclusion after my first two yoga classes in the gym. After all, I was able to take the class and make it all the way to the end without passing out. Therefore, *I was the shit,* as my kids would say.

I would have happily stayed with my gym forever had my first yoga teacher not abandoned me. This is how it feels when your yoga teacher leaves you; it is *abandonment.* This was a huge bummer, but it did serve to launch me into a bigger world of yoga.

My first yoga teacher was pretty in a sad way with brown hair and large, cheerless eyes. I could not tell if she was twenty-five or thirty-five. She was young, but she had a teenage child, so that kind of threw me off. She lived with her mother, who, I gathered, took care of the two of them in every way possible.

Every few weeks my teacher would disappear and the gym would get a sub. This probably should have alerted me, but I was so in love with my teacher's tattoos and piercings, her deep spiritual connection and her aura of detachment, that I never noticed she was just plain spacey. Concerned after the fifth disappearance in two months, I asked another class member, "Where did she go?"

"Rehab."

Huh? Here I am thinking that I had found my guru. She was amazing and so deeply connected to me. She showed me how to do Down Dog, *Adho Mukha Svanasana*. She would say, "Breathe" at just the exact moment I would breathe—*OMG!* She must have been a mind reader!

The last time I saw her, she had just returned from her latest disappearing act and took her seat at the front of the room. She sat down and then sagged back against the wall. She sort of smiled and her head flopped to the side. We began the practice.

"Down Dog," she said. We took our place on the mat.

"Right leg high," she said. Up it went.

"Knee to nose," she said. In it went.

"Right leg high," she said. Up it went.

"Knee to nose." In it went.

Her head was flopping from side to side keeping time like a metronome with our breath.

It continued like this for about twenty minutes. She never switched our legs. She never took us out of the Dog. I started to get worried, like, what if my leg falls off? But despite being older and wiser, despite being of sound mind and body, despite having been a *director of a $120 million company and the graduate of an Ivy League school*, I was too intimidated to stop this insanity. *"Michelle,"* I was screaming inside, *"Wake the fuck up."*

Then everything went silent. We looked over at her and she had passed out! She was completely unconscious with a little drool coming out of her mouth. A gentleman from a nearby mat went up to her and tried to shake her awake. Her head bobbed up and down. Her eyes flitted open and around in her head. She looked at us, smiled, drifted off to the right and went down for good.

It was time for a new yoga teacher.

The Journey Begins

Like many, I had started my yoga journey in the health club. I belonged to a gym where I could find a stationary bicycle, open up a book and semi-cycle myself into better shape. Truth be told, I turned the pages faster than I pedaled.

The club I found in Colorado offered yoga, and so, when I was looking to heal my back from a riding injury, it was the first place I went. The gym is the first place for many starter yogis, and not a bad place to begin. Often, gym yoga is free with the membership, and I know of many very fine yoga instructors who teach in health clubs. About 99% of new yoga students walk into the gym yoga class because they are in pain. And the other 1% are lost and are looking for the Pilates class. (That was me.)

Yet, just a few months into yoga I was hooked. While my back had improved, my spirits were also incredibly light. And much to my husband's delight, rather than spending my limited free time in the mall, I was practicing headstands in our bedroom.

"This is the most affordable insane thing you've ever done," he said.

And then my teacher passed out. So while the club looked around for another spiritual guide, I looked around for another yoga studio. In retrospect, I probably needed to be tossed out of a very comfortable nest.

I didn't have to look far. In Colorado, second only to California for yoga practiced per capita, the studios are like Starbucks. There is one on every corner. The first studio I found offered Power Yoga and hot Bikram Yoga, the two fastest growing trends in America. Both forms revived yoga from becoming an ancient dying art.

The Power practice, or a heated athletic Vinyasa Yoga style, is very appealing to Americans. The students perform yoga poses while the teacher says things like, "You are strong. You are powerful. Let go of your shit and get out of your way." It is a venti serving of pop culture psychology and pushups. And it is fun.

However, the name Power Yoga is a misnomer for yoga, because at some point everyone becomes stuck in their practice, and you realize that although yoga may be powerful, it is also equally humbling. I wonder if the class had been called "Powerless Yoga," would it have been as popular? Or called the "Cit Happens" studio? But I digress.

When I left the gym and walked into my first yoga studio, I was excited to be in a "real" yoga studio. It smelled slightly sweaty and smoky with incense. There were lots of little outfits you could buy if your "girls" were still where they were supposed to be, and your stomach hadn't been home to two boys. The teachers were mostly tattooed and pierced, and after I put my mat down I noticed tiny ants scurrying around, which I thought must be extremely authentic. I was in Heaven. By then, I had been practicing for almost two years at the health club and thinking, you know, I was pretty good. So I found a spot at the front of the room. *Check me out, you yoga bitches!*

That class turned out to be the most humiliating hour of my life, and that's including childbirth. I had no idea what they were doing. What the hell was "*Parsvakonasana*? They might as well have been saying "pickapeckofpickledfreakingpeppers-asana." What had my gym class teacher been teaching me? I had never seen these poses before in my life!

And that is how I opened the door to the Asana Bank.

More Than Human Tricks

From the first day, I was captivated. Some of these people were like crazy circus performers pressing into Headstand, *Sirsasana,* balancing on their arms stretching into the splits. I was spellbound. Who are these people? I couldn't even touch my toes. I had been practicing for nearly two years and nobody told me you were supposed to straighten your legs. What on earth had my first yoga teacher been teaching me?

Like a fish jumping for a fly, those first few years in a real yoga studio I was going hard and fast after the new poses. At first I practiced once or twice a week. Then it became five or six times. Every time I went to my mat it was to learn something new—another new posture, another new variation. I became an addict to innovation. I did not want to spend time on a pose I thought I knew. I only wanted to conquer something challenging. Who wanted to do Downward Facing

Dog, *Adho Mukha Svanasana*? Ugh. Bring on Headstand, *Sirsasana*, baby. In fact, if I went to a class and a teacher did not show me a new pose, I left disappointed. Hah, I thought, I am soooooo much better than that class. If I did not find something I could not do, I felt ripped off.

Months into my new yoga practice, I was deep into making deposits into the Asana Bank of yoga. Every new day brought a new pose for the bank. If I could do Crow, *Bakasana*, could I do it with one leg extended? *Cha Ching!* If I could do Revolved Crescent Lunge, *Parivrtta Anjaneyasana*, could I do it binding my arms? *Cha Ching!* And let's not even talk about inversions. Over and over again I propped myself against the back of the room, and I flopped my legs in the air like throwing spaghetti against a wall. Someday, I hoped, it would stick. But the challenge kept me going.

People spend varying amounts of time pursuing the Asana Bank, making more and more deposits that will start to yield less and less returns. I spent about eight years there, but I am not a fast learner. I thought that the more postures I could do, the "better" I was at yoga. But it turned out I was wrong.

If you blindly pursue the Asana Bank long enough, one of three things will occur:

- You will hit a plateau.
- You will become injured.
- You will get older and the body will fail you.

Trust me, if the first two don't happen, the third one will get you every time. In my case, all three possibilities got me at once. I realized that after years and years of practice

I was no closer to opening my hamstrings than I ever was. I had sciatica from trying so hard to touch my toes. And performing a Handstand was as likely as winning the lottery. In fact, once I knocked myself out trying. That is when I asked myself, what am I doing here?

"When you finally ask yourself, why am I doing this," said the Ashtanga teacher David Swenson in a workshop I attended in New York, "then the yoga begins."

Yoga Is What You Feel, Not What You Can Do

At first, the pain in my rear was just that, an annoying pain in my rear. It was one, huge wake-up call. Soon the pain migrated down my leg. Then, the pain became unbearable when I was driving; my whole leg would throb and I would have to pull over the car to stretch. When it woke me up at night, I knew I had to see my super-handsome doctor. This man truly is the upside of aging.

"Sciatica," he said, looking at my hip and leg. "Maybe you should try yoga."

Other injuries got me as well, but nothing floored me like aging. I have osteoarthritis just about everywhere, and soon I realized that I was popping Advil to get through a yoga class. That is so messed up.

If it hurts, it's not yoga.

It took me some time to realize that the Asana Bank had messed me up. Pursuing the loud, showy part of yoga was not actually yoga. The poses teach us from the inside out, regardless of how the thing looks on the outside.

Help came from the acclaimed international yoga teacher, Desiree Rumbaugh.

In 2007, I was limping from sciatica and probably addicted to painkillers. I went looking for classes to take at a nearby yoga conference in Estes Park, Colorado. Although I usually sign up for the classes called, *"Advanced Experts Extreme Yoga: Additional Release Forms and a Power of Attorney Required,"* there was one called, *"Yoga Shouldn't Hurt: Help for the Lower Body."* It couldn't have spoken to me any louder than if it had been called, *"Michelle, Take This Workshop and Do Yourself a Favor."*

I put my mat in the middle of a room of 300 people who apparently, also couldn't bend over without screaming pain. But despite the size of the room, I believed Desiree was speaking directly to me. Every word she spoke went directly to my heart. We only did about five postures in two and a half hours, but each one completely changed my practice. I realized I no longer had to muscle into the poses. I could find the subtle places deep within even the simplest poses to open up and yield a new understanding between me and my body. Up until now, I had been at war with my body. Desiree showed me the way to find peace with myself.

On a New Path: Going Inside

From that conference, I found a new path: Alignment Yoga. I still enjoy Power Yoga today, because frankly, it is fun. I get a good sweat, it does not involve a running bra, and it gets me out of my *freaking head*, which goes non-stop most of the time. Flowing in Vinyasa Yoga means you don't know where you are going. The teacher is in charge; believe me, it's nice to relinquish control once in awhile when you are working, running two households and managing teenagers' lives. But truthfully, my heart belongs to yoga that is aligned. Every year on my mat, the Power practice gets a little harder on my body, and if you party hard on the mat, beware, you will have to be able to walk in the morning. Being aligned helps me feel better on the mat.

We don't know why we are drawn to certain teachers, or why we find ourselves in certain places at certain times in our lives. I believe it is fate and that our teachers are chosen for us. Sometimes we need to just go with it. From this conference, I was led to Amy Ippoliti.

So, after studying alignment for just a few months, I enrolled in an Immersion with Amy. This is a 108-hour intensive course, which meant for sure that my family would not be getting dinner from me for at least three weeks. The course changed my life and now I follow Amy around whenever I can. I kind of yoga-stalk her, and it would be creepy, except that when you fall in love with a teacher, that is what you do; you yoga-stalk them and it's okay.

From the Immersion, I discovered a new way of practicing yoga. Instead of going just for a pose, we went for the feeling as well. Instead of focusing only on our bodies, we also focused on our hearts. We went inside first, and then the physical practice seemed to come together.

To this day, I credit Amy with saving not just my yoga practice, but in many aspects, my life. She taught me how to practice yoga so that I could restore my mobility and get rid of my pain. She encouraged me to try again, and again, even when I doubted myself. In so many ways, my story owes its telling to her. She helped me find my attitude, and my "inner badass," so I could grow better as I got older. And it was on my mat, in her class, that I decided to write again after many years of struggling to find my voice.

Yoga Is From the Inside Out

Being in alignment changed not only my practice, but first and foremost my attitude. The Asana Bank became an empty account. Instead of looking for teachers who demonstrated pretty poses and then said, "Your turn," I began to seek out teachers who could help me touch my toes. If I stayed in Down Dog, *Adho Mukha Svanasana* for the rest of my life, but actually got it right, I would be happy. The joy was in the details, in the tiniest realization of my hamstrings lengthening or my hips opening. I knew that if there was something I could not do, there was probably an answer on my mat. I only had to persevere to find it.

"Being an advanced student is not being loud," explained Iyengar teacher Jason Crandall in a class in Estes Park. "It's being subtle."

I was taking a class with Jason on how to keep your composure when you are near the edge in a pose. His point is that being an advanced student is not chasing new poses at every opportunity, but finding how all the parts work together. "It is like a fine wine," he said, "aging the various tones and subtle flavors until something brilliant emerges." It's listening to something inside of you that tells you where to go.

I knew that before I could grow my practice in any meaningful way, I needed to heal myself first. It took a year, but I healed my sciatica completely. Then I turned my attention to my back, which had twenty percent curvature of the spine from osteoporosis. I was all hunched up and it was ruining my backbends. (What backbends, really? I had no practice in the "heart openers" whatsoever.) So I addressed my shoulders and upper back with daily stretching. I would lie on a block for twenty minutes at a time. I would work my shoulders open before every practice. I was obsessed, but this time it was with the right thing.

To Move Ahead, Go Back to the Beginning

"The Primary Series is very important," David Swenson told us in a workshop on Long Island. "The Secondary Series is a little important," Swenson continued. "The Third through Fifth Series are just for show."

It is true for any style of yoga.

The beginner series is where you will learn the most.

Everything you need to know in order to do the most advanced pose is in the first class you ever took. Actually, it is probably in Downward Facing Dog, *Adho Mukha Svanasana*.

Two years after my first Immersion, I met Amy in January 2009 for an advanced teacher's practice. "What posture do you want to work on this year?" she asked us. Amy believes that if you do not set goals, you won't reach them. Some people wanted to move from Handstand, *Adho Mukha Vrksasana*, into *Eka Pada Koundinyasana II*, Hurdlers, without touching the ground. Some wanted *Eka Pada Viparita Dandasana*, which is a one-legged variation of Wheel Pose. When it was my turn, I told the truth.

"*Bhujangasana*," I said. "Cobra Pose."

Amy looked at me puzzled. This is a very basic pose; in fact, one of the first you learn in a yoga class, and surely even a nincompoop would have learned it in 108 hours of being in her classroom. But in actuality, it's hard to get right if you have rounded shoulders and a back tighter than a drum. The pose requires strength in the lower body to secure the sacrum and to enable the upper body to rise. You need to keep the wrists and forearms spiraled inward, while the upper arms simultaneously roll outward. The shoulder blades need to

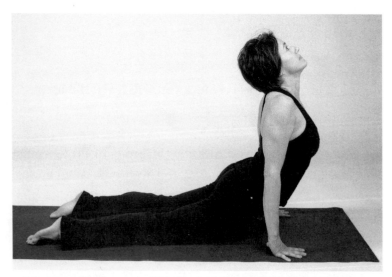

Cobra Pose, *Bhujangasana*. This "beginner" pose is still the hardest for me.

come down and root on the back, and then very subtly, the chest lifts and expands like the fan of a cobra's head.

"What about Handstand?" she suggested. "What about Dropbacks (when you drop from standing into a Wheel behind you)?" After all, I was moving into what some would consider an early intermediate practice by then.

"Nope, I'll be good with Cobra," I replied.

Here's the reason why. I have no doubt that if I had picked any advanced pose, I might have gotten there. But the pursuit of the Asana Bank at that time fed a part of my ego that did not need feeding. I know Amy could take me anywhere I want to go, then and now. But where I needed to go was back to the beginning. I needed to open up my shoulders and get a stronger core before I tried anything crazy again. I needed to continue to assess my practice in the here and now, before going into the unknown.

I figured *Bhujangasana* would teach me these lessons. And then a funny thing happened to me while I was concentrating on Cobra Pose that year. My practice exploded. I was able to straighten my arms with a near perfect vertical rise in Upward Facing Dog, *Urdhva Mukha Svanasana*. I could suddenly touch my toes after trying for ten years. And I was just about down to the floor in the Splits Pose, *Hanumanasana*.

How could this happen? I had stopped chasing the pose, and instead I focused on the actions I needed to cultivate. I stopped attending intermediate yoga classes and went back to the beginner series. Instead of focusing on what I couldn't do, I focused on what I could, and it made all the difference.

It was perseverance that brought me to a new understanding with my practice. Rather than turning up the volume pose after pose, I started cultivating the tranquility inside. I wanted to know *me* better, to know what I needed, and to give it to myself as an act of love. My practice has become so much more vibrant by doing less. Now I look at yoga poses and understand the baby steps involved. I see everything as an opportunity to go back to the beginning and find the pieces that lead to the pose. In turn, I grow a little better from the inside out. I measure my success with each breath, or with each tiny fraction I am able to stretch, or by each muscle I am able to engage. That is growing better with yoga, realizing that the more you practice, the less you know, and being willing to go back and learn again.

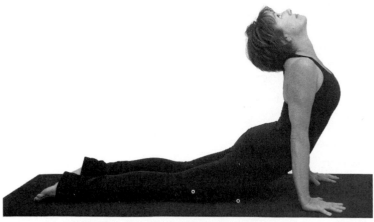

Cobra 2014. We change with practice and patience.

A Lesson From the Mat

How to Improve Your Long Game

A funny thing happened to my husband one summer. He went to a Golf Pro to improve his long game. And in the end, he improved his short game.

I also wanted to improve my long game. When I first started yoga, I was frantically pursuing the big moves: the arm rotation in Half Pigeon, *Eka Pada Rajakapotasana*; Handstand, *Adho Mukha Vrksasana* in the middle of the room; Upward Facing Wheel, *Urdhva Dhanurasana*, without shoulder pain. I wanted the full splits, *Hanumanasana*, without tearing my groin apart. So I kept hitting the advanced practices in town, and taking classes from the hardest teachers, and watching everything from the back of the room. My practice didn't improve, but I became very adept at "*Watch-asana*."

It wasn't until I took a giant step backwards that I improved my practice. The year I focused on the fundamentals is the year my practice moved forward. And for the first time, I understood how to get where I wanted to go by improving the building blocks of yoga and not necessarily going for the big pose.

A Lesson From the Mat

How to Improve Your Short Game

Do the advanced poses teach the yoga principles? Or does knowing the yoga principles get you to the advanced poses? The answer to the latter is yes.

The advanced poses are there to pull you out of alignment. So you need to work harder to stay in alignment. To do the hardest poses, you need to become an expert at the fundamentals or the short game.

Here are some guidelines to improving your practice:

- Work on the fundamentals over and over again because the brain has a way of forgetting and the body has habits that need to be overcome.

- Recognize that yoga is humbling. Stop and think: Where am I stuck? Then put aside the pose you really want and find the most basic pose that can get you there.

- First things first: Concentrate on standing up straight with shoulders back and tummy in, straightening your legs when folding forward, engaging your muscles, engaging your core, and so on. You cannot do the "advanced" poses until you are advanced in the beginning poses.

- Be relentless. You will not get what you want by whining. You will get it by practicing every day. Yes. Every. Single. Day.

A Lesson From the Mat

Be Who You Are

Yoga is humbling. Not achieving certain poses has taught me more about life than the poses I can easily do. We become better from the challenges, not the effortless stuff.

Chasing the most glorious yoga poses is a lot like trying to be the biggest and best that you can be, when in fact, yoga teaches us to be happy with who we are, at that moment. It is always a balance between *tapas*, or the desire to be better, and *santosha*, the contentment with who we are and what we have. I've learned to aim for the balance. If all I can do today is Downward Facing Dog, *Adho Mukha Svanasana*, then I will do it brilliantly. I do not need to go to the splits to get validation. However, I will continue to practice in order to do the splits someday. If you can be who you are, and be happy with it, yet still hold out hope for living better in the future, then you are living brilliantly.

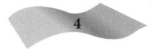

Travel Often, Pack Light

It is better to travel well than to arrive.

~ Buddha

Yoga is the perfect vacation for the agoraphobic. You can go where you want, and never have to leave home.

I know what it is to leave home. My mother, bless her heart, is a serial mover. I counted eighteen different homes, including living on a boat, before I graduated from high school; eighteen different apartments between New York and Florida. Eighteen times I had to pack up my Barbies, put everything in a box, leave friends, and make friends. There were some moves where I didn't have time to unpack. Then just when I thought it was safe to hang my picture of Bobby Sherman, we were off again.

In addition to the moving, my parents were divorced, so I divided my childhood between my mother's apartment—wherever we were—and my father's on Park Avenue. Back and forth, back and forth. To be divorced was to be divided. I was constantly on the move.

It is no wonder that today I am something of an agoraphobic.

A functioning agoraphobic, that's what I am.

I try not to make a big deal of it, so I guess that makes me a semi-functioning agoraphobic who pretends to be a good traveler in life.

This is what happens when I get ready to leave the house: I start sweating. I feel my heart pounding. I get extremely nervous and agitated. Then I have a fight with my husband. This works like a charm. Once we start bickering with each other, I am happy to leave the house and forget that I am an agoraphobic at heart who at one point wanted to stay home with her crabby husband.

When we were first married and had to pack for a trip, like say, our honeymoon, Mike noticed that I would go into a full-on panic attack two weeks before our departure. This would result in a fourteen-day fight until the night before we left, when I would dissolve in a messy puddle of scotch and soda.

After a few trips, he put two and two together, and the answer was he'd pour me a double and then would do all the packing. The problem was I'd arrive wherever we were going and didn't have any bras. Or jeans. Or, we'd be going to the beach and I wouldn't have a bathing suit, which I took as a sign from the Universe that I shouldn't be wearing one in public. After awhile, I realized I had to get functioning again and pack for myself.

You would think that moving so many times in child-hood would get me used to it, like a bird that heads south in the winter over and over again, but that's not the way it works. When you have no roots, when you lack stability, you want *more* of it, not less. It was this yearning for permanence in my life that finally got me over my fear of leaving the house. Yoga was bringing me more stability on my mat, and it was my desire to go deeper into the practice that finally got me out of my little world.

The Suburban Seduction

Today I live in suburbia and here is the thing about the suburbs: You never, *ever* have to leave. You could live your entire life inside a five-mile radius and be completely happy.

In the suburbs, we have schools, Starbucks and a mortuary; it's the circle of life.

Although by nature a city mouse, I moved to the suburbs for the kids. When my oldest was born, we rented a very cool townhouse in Santa Monica, California. But taking him to a park meant loading the baby, the car seat, stroller, a diaper bag the size of a small steamer trunk, and snacks to sustain life for a month into our tiny hatchback for an hour drive in traffic so he could sit on a small patch of grass in the sun. *OMG!* Who wouldn't be an agoraphobic?

Then we moved into a 1,800 square foot slice of heaven off of Mulholland Drive in Los Angeles. Our first home was on the top of a hill with the San Fernando Valley stretched out beneath us. In the evenings we would stand at the edge of the lawn watching the city lights twinkle below. At Christmastime, when the boys were little, we'd point to the lights of a passing jet landing at Burbank Airport, and say, "There goes Santa on his sleigh."

When my sons were toddlers, I still worked in an office in Santa Monica and said goodbye everyday to the husband, the nanny, the maid, and the boys as I courageously made my way downtown to work with the grownups and occasionally have lunch in Beverly Hills. Then after going through four nannies in two years, and being stranded at airports in bad weather across the country, Mike and I realized this was not working for us. Someone had to be home; we decided it would be me.

I was quickly seduced by the San Fernando Valley. I spent my days shuttling the kids from park to park, making pottery and attending Mommy & Me music and art classes. I'd meet my fellow post-working mothers at any number of local kid-friendly restaurants for lunch, and then head home for naptime. I trusted the kids were really napping as I lay passed out on the couch.

I was so happy never leaving a five-mile radius that you wouldn't know I used to be a New Yorker! Although I would occasionally take the kids to a museum or to a park farther away, getting out of the neighborhood began to be harder and harder. I could not care less that a world existed outside my own. I was good.

But then something woke me up. It was called First Grade. The cost of private elementary school for both my boys was going to be $50,000 a year. That's a whole lot of lattes I would not be able to afford. Just about that time I flew to see my grandmother in Florida, and being a terrible flyer (of course, because I'm only a semi-functional agoraphobic), I outlined a plan for Mike in case my plane went down. He needed to know who he should marry next because there was no way he'd be able to keep up the toddlers' schedule of Mommy & Me classes and work at the same time.

"You don't have to worry about it if your plane goes down," Mike said to me. "I have a plan."

"You do?" I asked.

"Yes, of course. I'm going to get us out of here."

And just like that we realized that neither of us really wanted to be in California. So we moved to Colorado. We bought a book that was called something like, "The Best Places You Could Live in the World," and Boulder was rated very high. So we flew there first, looked around, and I had a heart attack.

"What is *with* the silver jewelry and the Earth shoes?" I asked the realtor at lunch on Pearl Street, the hub of all things hippy in town. "I'm a *freaking* brunette from New York. Tell me, is there a Tiffany's in this state?"

"Is she serious?" the realtor asked my husband.

"Completely," Mike said.

So the realtor pointed us toward the south and that is how we found Denver, where there were good schools, mountains for skiing, and (I'm happy to say) a Tiffany's nearby. And again we chose a suburban home for the convenience factor. Even the mall is less than three miles away. Life gets busy, the babies grow up, and one day you realize you haven't actually left your neighborhood in something like five years. I was a happy little agoraphobic pig in poo, let me tell you.

That is when my very comfortable daily routine of kids, breakfast, yoga, kids, lunch, sports, activities, dinner, homework, bedtime kind of blew up because my yoga teacher at the gym passed out. Once I was thrown out of the nest, I began to find more yoga in my 'hood, and then more yoga just slightly beyond my 'hood, and then one thing led to another, and one day I said to Mike, "Hey, maybe I'll become a yoga teacher."

But that is really what happened. I was content, and then I decided I wanted more. It might have been an extra strong triple venti from the suburban Starbucks. Or it was just something about yoga that really spoke to me. But one day, I thought, hey, what if I went to yoga teacher training school and learned more?

So I looked for a yoga teacher training program near my house, but as luck would have it, there were none. I realized that location is not the way one should pick out a school, much less a guru.

**Geography is only that, geography.
It is not a map for one's life.**

How Much Do You Want It?

Here is the thing about getting out of the house, or the neighborhood, or moving past anything that frightens you terribly: *You have to really want it.* You have to want it more than the thing that's holding you back. And I really wanted to know more about yoga. I wanted to go deeper on my mat. I wanted more out of the "rinse and repeat" of my life. So fighting the fear in my heart, I signed up for my first yoga teacher training program at a studio in downtown Denver, about eighteen miles away. I was able to sign up on the phone so I wouldn't have to leave my house. But when the reality hit that my new school was *eighteen miles away from home*, I went into the bathroom and threw up. How was I ever going to get there?

After whining for a week to Mike that I made a terrible, 200-hour, $2,000 mistake, he had enough. He put me into the car and drove the route to show me how easy it was going to be to get there. He made a map, timed the drive, and practically threw me out the door on my first day of school.

In addition to a husband who knows when I need to be thrown out of the house, I have a girlfriend who was thrilled to hear I was doing something so completely insane. If something sounds insane, she is ready to sign up. This woman is my idol. She is an adventurer. She's been to every continent (seriously), travels abroad at least three times a year and has brought her children along since they were out of diapers. (You couldn't pay me a million dollars to take my children on a sixteen-hour plane ride until the electronic game things were invented.)

She is one of the most daring people I know. She skis the steeps, she scubas the deeps, and she hasn't met a horse she couldn't ride. When everybody else thought I was crazy to go to yoga school, she promised to go to as many classes as she could with me. When I doubted myself, she gave me confidence. When I had to practice four hours a day, and then go to school for four more hours at night, she said she was jealous. (Liar!) When I cried that if I took anymore Advil, I'd test positive for an illegal substance, she was there on the mat next to me urging me on. But the best part was when I had to try a new class or a new teacher in a new studio, often she would find the time to come with me, which helped me with many of my old agoraphobic fears.

Then one day the curriculum required me to take an Iyengar class downtown, in a very strange part of the city, where there were factories and warehouses and not much else other than this little studio. I was a bit afraid, so I called to pick up my yoga BFF, but she balked at the inner city locale as well.

**It seems that no matter how adventurous we are,
or how fearless our heart,
there can be a boundary real or imagined.
This is the edge of our zip code.**

"I'm sorry," she said when I gave her the address. "I love you, but that's too far out of my zip code."

Travel Often, See New Things

The zip code is like suburbia; it is comfortable. It is warm and safe inside, and just a little scary outside. Inside the zip code, we have our favorite restaurants, our favorite movie theaters and shops and schools. We like our home the way it is with the worn-out rugs, we have our comfortable sweater that really should not be worn in public. We seal ourselves in a bubble because it is comfortable. We stop trying new things and making new friends. There is a reluctance to travel out of our zip code.

The same is true in yoga. The tendencies toward "good enough" become noticeable. After going through an initial adventurous stage, some yogis draw a boundary around them past which they will not venture. Some hide behind their school of yoga ("I only practice Ashtanga..."). Others claim the ubiquitous neck injury so they cannot do Headstand, *Sirsasana*. (Honestly, does anyone out there *not* have a neck injury?) I also like the "I can't do core exercises because I just had a baby" excuse, even when the "baby" has celebrated his 15th birthday. (I just used that one the other day.)

People, it's time to let this stuff go.

Your Bag Weighs Less When You Let Stuff Go

We are lighter when we unpack. About fifteen years ago, my mother started giving things away. Of course, you are wondering, how could she have that much with all the moving? But my mother is plucky and determined, so each time she moved there would be a semi-tractor trailer filled with a lifetime of memories following along behind her.

At first, I received a string of pearls given to her on her sixteenth birthday. And then a cocktail ring arrived by registered mail. Slowly the furniture started making an appearance. It came couch by couch, a bookcase, a painting. And then one day, a huge moving van pulled up and out rolled my mother's entire life.

"Have you lost your mind?" I asked when I reached her on the phone.

"On the contrary," she replied happily, "I think I found it!"

My mother is a modern day gypsy who is always ready for the next adventure. Wherever we lived, I took comfort that home was where she and the antiques were. The homes would change, but the stuff always stayed the same. It turned out that all that stuff had been weighing her down.

When I asked her what she was going to sit on now that I had the sofa, she replied she had no time to sit! Furthermore, she was going to redecorate in "Scandinavian Modern," which I think means plywood. She was delighted with the change.

"I had no idea how much that stuff had been holding me back," she said. "I feel like I've lost 100 pounds." Actually, it was probably closer to 1,500 pounds.

**Our stuff weighs us down and holds us back.
It might be time to let it go.**

We get trapped by the memories and guilt. If you are surrounded by clutter, then you are likely surrounded by fear. Fear of throwing something away even if it's useless, is fear of parting with the past. Keeping things you don't use is fear of the future not being able to provide. Living in the moment, using only what you need, is living without fear and with a belief in abundance.

Holding onto stuff is holding onto a kind of security blanket. Take my closet, for instance. It used to be filled with a ton of clothes that no longer fit me after two pregnancies. Then one day I realized I had nothing to wear. I was so disgusted that I had been clinging to this illusion of being four sizes smaller than I was, that I grabbed armfuls of clothing and threw them out. My husband came home from work and had a heart attack.

"Honey, we've been robbed," he yelled from upstairs.

"We haven't been robbed."

"Then where are all your clothes?"

"I donated what didn't fit, and that's what's left," I told him.

"Holy cow," he said, "You need to go shopping."

OH MY GOD! Letting go was working better than I had imagined.

When the stuff piles so high that you can't move or grow, then it's time to get rid of the stuff. Easy, when it's a closet of jeans. Not so easy, when you can't see what's holding you back.

If you want to be filled up with something new, you must unpack your bags and clean out your closets.

You have to let go of your stories, your hang-ups, and your issues. Then you can fill up with new hope. If you think you can't do something, you won't. But if you put that thought aside, you might be astounded with the possibilities.

I am never more content, more complete, or more open to possibility than when I am simply alone with my mat. Yet I had to let go of my agoraphobia to get there.

The Unexpected Adventures

The best adventures in life often don't come with a GPS, or a map, or even very much baggage. They often come out of nowhere. Sometimes the unexpected adventures are the ones that put us right where we are supposed to be.

When I was about ten years old, I took an adventure that changed my life. My father had arranged a vacation for us on a friend's private island in the Caribbean. At the last minute something happened to the reservations, I'm not sure what, but my seat on the airline disappeared. My mother wasn't going to let me miss this vacation, so she booked another ticket for me that required a change in Miami, and then a night in Jamaica where I would wait for my father to take me to the island the next day.

In my mother's excitement to give me a nice vacation, she did not consider that it might have been insane to send a ten year old alone to Jamaica. But nothing stops my mother, so bright and early in the morning she kissed me goodbye at Kennedy airport and gave me $25 for emergencies. In Miami, the airline representative helped me to change planes. Landing in Jamaica, the customs agent greeted me at the counter and asked for my passport. How many ten year olds have a passport? I offered the only identification I had—my N.Y.C. library card! Apparently, not many drug dealers try to enter Jamaica on a library card, so minutes later the hotel representative was whisking me off to paradise.

At the hotel, I was booked into the Royal Palm Suite, which apparently comes with your own personal body-guard when you are just ten years old and travelling alone. I changed into my prettiest pink dress and floated downstairs to the lobby where the largest, blackest man I had ever seen was waiting for me. *Cha Ching!* I knew instantly I had hit the lottery.

He bowed and kissed my hand. I had knee socks on and my skinny little legs were shaking! I'd seen plenty of African American men in New York. After all, I lived in Greenwich Village, but this man was the color of perfect ebony, and his chest was massive! He wore a pale grey suit with a white shirt that showed off his deep color even more. He smiled at me and introduced himself. I knew at that moment that even though I was being raised in a lesbian community, I definitely wasn't gay.

He spent the rest of the evening catering to my every whim. (Oh, what a terrible way to be introduced to the wonders of men, with a false reality that this is how they will treat you for the rest of your life!) We ate dinner and danced to the hotel reggae band. My prince requested the band play "Michelle," by the Beatles, and he danced with me until I got too tired to stay on my feet. Then he picked me up like the feather I was, and carried me around the dance floor. I was smitten. At one point he asked me if I missed my parents very much, and I was like, "Who?" Around midnight he walked me to my room, and outside the door, he bent down very low, thanked me for a magical evening "Miss Michelle," placed my little hand in his and kissed it again. I think that may have been my first spontaneous orgasm.

To this day, the sound of reggae music brings back this adventure that led me across the threshold from sheltered child to independent young woman. I had no idea where I was going. I had no GPS, or map, or even a passport. I did not yet fear leaving home.

In the space of one day, I was changed.
I was fearlessly thrilled with the unknown.

As we get older, the unknown gets scarier. There are still days when I am afraid to leave my house. I've got anxiety meds, and I've got yoga. But I can also go back to this incredible place for me, where I remember that even when I might be lost, it could be that I'm exactly where I'm supposed to be, whether I know it or not.

A Lesson From the Mat

Get Out of Your Zip Code!

Signs you may be stuck in your zip code on the mat:

Being resistant to change. You have a rigid schedule. Monday is the noon class with Tom, Tuesday is the 5:30 P.M. with Dick, and Wednesday is the 8:30 A.M. with Harry. The irony is that the student believes she is practicing with the "best" teachers and therefore getting the "best" instruction. But in fact, she is only getting the same instruction and closing herself off from new guidance.

Being resistant to guidance. If a teacher offers you an adjustment, and you think any of the following, you might be stuck:
- This feels weird, it has to be wrong.
- I know how to practice yoga, back off!
- My teacher told me to do it *this* way.
- *Who is this bitch?*

Being resistant to other styles of yoga. You've chosen your favorite kind of yoga and now you never try anything else. Wrong! You can learn something from everyone. Unpack the expectations from your bag. I know a couple who went to a yoga retreat in Costa Rica. On their return, they said the resort was beautiful, but the yoga was not very good. I asked why not? They said it wasn't "Power Yoga," just some other kind. It is hard to imagine that any kind of yoga on the beach could be disappointing. When this happens, it is generally not about the yoga, but about your expectations. Try to let that go when you pack your bag.

It is rumored that in 2005 when Mr. Iyengar was eighty-six and he visited the United States, he tried a Vinyasa class with music in Estes Park, Colorado and announced that it was "marvelous fun." All I'm saying is it was a rumor, but I believe it.

One of the biggest awakenings I ever received was in an Iyengar class in Paris. I was on vacation and only had a limited time during the day to practice. So I ran to the nearest yoga studio on the Left Bank and took whatever was being offered. Wouldn't you know it, the teacher was a Goddess. I remember Maryam to this day. Her instruction, mostly in French, was like a laser beam to my practice. She honed in on my shoulders and recognized immediately that the right was different from the left. The adjustments she made and the instruction she gave me has stayed with me to this day. What I would have missed had I only looked for my regular style of yoga in a language I could understand!

Being resistant to being uncomfortable. Yoga is like a crazy fox. When it gets easy, you have stopped practicing. When it gets hard, you are on the path. Remember, *yoga not easy*. Contentment, *santosha*, is necessary to find peace. However, contentment could also be a way to mask a lack of initiative. You may be at ease saying you do not want to do a Handstand in the middle of the room. I know my mother, for example, has no desire whatsoever to do a Handstand anywhere, anytime. And she is very content, very happy to say so. But, if you really, secretly, desire to do a Handstand, then you must go for it. This is growing better. This is not giving up on your wild heart.

Getting out of our comfort zone might take us to new places that in turn, make us better in the long run. And if everyone was able to live a better life, the world would be a happier place, and we agoraphobics wouldn't be afraid to leave home.

A Lesson From the Mat

Pack Light

Some of us have a lot of stuff; the older we get, we accumulate more. We need to be diligent, keeping only what serves us and discarding everything else that gets in our way such as:

- **The mind.** If your mind is telling you "noooooo," thank it for contributing and move on. The mind is like a child that sometimes does not play well with others.
- **The past.** If you've fallen down in an inversion, hopefully, you've learned something and are now wiser to try again. Just because it happened in the past, it may not happen again in the present. There are no guarantees.
- **The patterns.** If you always get into a pose the same old way, try a new approach. Another variation might reveal something new.
- **Unpack before you travel again.** You have to let things go, so you can fill up with new. Meditate. Make peace with the past, and you might be astounded with the possibilities of the present.

A Lesson From the Mat

Turn off the GPS

How to deal with being lost:
The truth is, we often don't know where we are, or where we are going. Yet this is where yoga begins. Yoga is partly about becoming more comfortable with the unknown. That is one reason to try new poses and new variations.

How to get comfortable with being lost:
- **Acknowledge the moment.** Recognize that you may not be completely lost, you are only temporarily out of your zip code. Most misalignments are temporary.
- **Identify the familiar.** In the novelty of a new pose, practice what you do know: the basic principles. And remember to breathe. The way home starts with the breath.
- **Recognize that the GPS is a pretense.** You may think you are on a charted course, but in fact, you are constantly travelling to new territory. In the biggest picture, we are *matter* on a planet hurtling a million miles an hour through space. So relax and enjoy the ride.
- **Open your eyes.** When you look at the GPS, you see a picture of the world. But when you look out the window, you see the world itself. When you look at a yoga pose, see if you can observe not just the shape, but also the quality of the heart and the principles involved.

- **Step back to step in.** On the GPS, there is a button that allows you to see the picture from far away. When you feel a little lost, step back and take in the whole scene. This is tapping into the bigger picture, or the Universal energy.

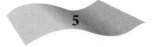

Be a Beginner, Always

I have come to a point in my life
where there is nothing more important to me,
than my own growth.
~ Baron Baptiste, *Journey Into Power*

I used to ride racehorses.

I know this sounds crazy, but I wouldn't lie because there are too many ways for you to find out if I'm lying, and then Oprah will not invite me to her show someday as an example of a middle-aged woman who teaches yoga, has raised children, and who used to ride racehorses.

In 1987, I rode at the Birmingham Turf Club, a multi-million dollar racetrack in Alabama, where I was also a reporter on the afternoon newspaper. It's sad to note that both businesses are gone today. The newspaper went under like so many across America and the racetrack is now home to greyhounds. However I'm still here with the memories.

Back then, in my twenties, I'd start my day by making my way to the track in the early mornings with a steaming cup of coffee balanced on the dashboard. There is nothing like seeing the sun rising over Alabama's dusty red clay earth. That dirt clings to everything like a lacy red shroud. It used to stick to my boots and I'd find it on my skirts as well. I still carry a bit of it with me now.

Like every jock, my day started with peeing in a cup to prove there was nothing more addictive in my system than coffee and chocolate. Then I'd head over to the barn to be weighed in front of a dozen men who were often lighter than me. That's humbling. Finally, I'd see which horse I was exercising that day.

It wasn't that I was a great rider (although I'm not bad), or a "horse whisperer," or even a good luck charm. I happened to be the right weight and in the right place at the right time. It also helped that I used to be one crazy ass girl. Trainers like to exercise their horses ten pounds heavier than they ride in a race, and way back when in that Alabama summer, I was just tipping the scales at about ten pounds heavier than the jocks. *(You thought I was going to tell my weight. Are you insane?)*

I made $15 a ride, and depending on my schedule, I could take about a half dozen thoroughbreds around the track before I needed to clean up for my day job. It was sweet money for something I loved. And although I only sort of knew what I was doing on the backs of those magnificent animals, it just didn't matter. I could hang on pretty good and the track supervisors on the quarter horses could catch me when I couldn't rein one in.

There is nothing quite like being a fledgling jockey or an exercise rider without any expectations that I would ride beautifully. I didn't have to be first or clear a fence with my mare's hooves tucked in and ears forward. If I could just hang on to those thoroughbreds and not get tossed into the dirt, it was a very good day. It got me to thinking:

What if we didn't have to become an expert at life?
What if we were always meant to be beginners?

At the racetrack there is a clear advantage to being a beginner. For the first year in a jockey's career, they get to "carry the bug," which means they will ride in a race ten pounds lighter than the other riders. This is a huge advantage. HUGE! Because any horse that rides lighter than the others can probably run faster in the race. The novice jocks are often the most sought after riders at the tracks.

Carry the Bug as Long as You Can

There is a saying in yoga: Beginners and advanced students are easy to teach because they BOTH *know* they know nothing. Intermediates are difficult because they think they know it all.

About five years into my yoga practice, I went to an Advanced/ Beginner level Iyengar class in Denver. The teacher asked each of us how long we've been practicing. The first said, "I have been practicing for several years, but I still have much to learn." He asked the second, and she replied that she had tried yoga a few times and was now an "intermediate." To which the teacher replied that he had been practicing for twenty-five years; studied with B.K.S. Iyengar and Sri K. Pattabhi Jois; that he had also spent two years in India, blah, blah, blah; and he still thought of himself as a beginner. Then he turned to me, and being a quick study, I said, "I've never practiced yoga before in my life!"

"Then how on earth did you get into this class?" he roared.

"The front desk put me here, sir, because they said you were the best teacher, and so I humbly place myself in your hands," I replied. Score one for Michelle.

The truth is every teacher is a student, and every student is a beginner. If you think you have the answers, you have only closed yourself off from learning more.

Yoga is, if nothing else, a lesson in humility. The more teachers I meet, the more I travel, the more seminars I take, the more I practice, the more I teach, the more I learn, the less I feel I know. Something new is revealed to me each time about yoga. It is endlessly revealing, and if I hoped to have all the answers, it would be endlessly maddening. But now, I have decided to be a student first, and always. I learned to "carry the bug" in yoga and be a novice for as long as I can.

Go Back to Start

The year I became a yoga teacher, and therefore back when I knew everything, I went to a yoga conference in Colorado and signed up for an advanced back-bending class with Desiree Rumbaugh. They call these poses "heart openers," but in reality, they were just spine-crackers to me. I had no business being in an "advanced" class for anything in those days, and secondly I was nothing close to being "backbend girl."

Nevertheless, my favorite teacher was teaching so I felt safe to simply watch if there was no freaking way I could do it. There were about forty people in the room including several yogis with a very strong practice. Desiree was leading us through a warm-up and a review of the fundamental principles when she suddenly stopped the class. Looking around the room, she announced, "Nobody here is ready for advanced heart openers. We are going to learn the basic principles of opening the shoulders instead."

Booooyah! That was new for me. I had never seen a teacher take her seat like that and put it on the line. You should have seen the faces on those mats! For me, it was a gift. And afterward, one of the strongest yogis in Colorado came up to me and confessed that he had learned more about backbends in that workshop by going over the fundamentals than ever before in his life.

"It changed my practice," he said.

"Me, too," I replied, although really, I didn't have much of a practice to begin with.

This is what I know for sure about yoga and life:

**If you don't know where you are in a pose,
go back to the basics.
Remember you are always a beginner at heart.**

The advanced poses become accessible to us because of our expertise with basic principles. The more advanced the pose, the more it will ask our bodies to go out of alignment. So, the crazier we get on the mat, the more diligent we must be about staying in the basic alignment. Whenever I am lost on my mat and scared that I am going to need Yoga 911, I say to myself, "Shins in, thighs back, scoop your tail, side body long, melt your heart, breathe." That is how I talk myself down from the edge.

A few years after Desiree's workshop, I attended a "One Day Immersion" in Denver with the founder of Power Yoga, Baron Baptiste. He surveyed the room of 400 and decided of all the powerful yogis in the room he was going to choose me to stand on my back. *Right?* I am not making this up because it is too easy for you to find out if I am telling the truth. Ask anyone in Colorado. Baron Baptiste came to town and picked a fifty-year-old woman to stand on her back in *Chaturanga*, Four-Limbed Staff Pose.

So while I held *Chaturanga* with arms bent in a low push up position as Baron stood on my back, I was not thinking I am an expert, I've got this in the bag. No, I was thinking the same thing over and over: side body long, head of the arm bones back, scoop your tail, breathe. Oh, I also thought, *"What the hell is he doing on my back?"* Yet he did it to prove a point—anyone can do these crazy poses. You just need to know the basic principles, and you need to believe you can.

Enjoy a Lack of Success

The beginner is honest. She knows she sucks at this. The first-time yogi approaches his mat with an open mind. He is thrilled to see his progress every day. Every adjustment is taken with eagerness to make a new change. Each suggestion is a doorway to improvement. The beginner is an empty vessel. He or she has no expectations. Every day is some new realization and a new achievement on the mat. In many ways, I was a better yogi, a truer student, when I knew myself to be a complete beginner and was wholly open to suggestion.

The practice of yoga truly begins, however, when all the initial excitement has worn off and you still can't reach

Kapotasana, King Pigeon Pose, or some other white whale of a pose that haunts your dreams. That's another way to tell that playtime is over and your practice has begun.

Years ago, when I decided to commit to teacher training, I thought yoga would be like anything else I had tried in my life—easy. I had been practicing for seven years and I thought this should be fun. You know, knock out a few classes, get my certificate, teach at the gym....

It didn't turn out to be that way. First of all, I was one of the oldest in the program, and spending eight hours a day sitting cross-legged on the floor nearly put me in rehab.

At graduation, I was shocked when I was not the first to be hired by the yoga studio. *Whaaat?* I had scored 100+ on my exam, acing even the bonus questions. And I was starting to acquire some very cute outfits. *Helloooooo?*

"Everyone is on a path," my mentor told me. "You will be there when you are ready."

I have never failed at anything (unless you count my first marriage, and possibly raising my children, and then there are a few of those pesky family relationships that could be a whole lot better). I regarded not being hired as a complete and utter condemnation of my perfect attendance at school, my perfect test scores, my perfect Warrior II, *Virabhadrasana II*. My husband, ever supportive, suggested that maybe I give this up and make dinner for a change.

Not completely deterred, I picked up a few corporate classes and a few privates from friends. Then I was hired by a gym that was obviously desperate for instructors, and from there I made my way into the studios. Somewhere in those first few months, I hurt a student with a bad adjustment. Not only was she hurt enough to have to lay off yoga for a few weeks, but I was devastated. No one goes into teaching yoga to hurt people.

I decided there might be a lesson here and I should not waste it. Maybe I wasn't ready? Perhaps I did not know enough to have people trust me with their bodies. I did not have the "answers." I was far from an expert. I was still a beginner. So in 2008, I went back to school.

This time I studied Anusara Yoga, known as an alignment-based and heart-oriented practice. It is also a system that can provide yoga therapy that can heal people, rather than cause more damage. Another Immersion, another teacher training, another year on Advil, and another year where my family did not have a hot meal. But the process of discovery has been endlessly revealing. And although the more I study, the less I feel I know, that is no longer endlessly maddening.

I am learning to enjoy the feeling of not knowing it all.

My teacher, Amy Ippoliti, says that if you make yourself a vessel, then the teachings can enter you more easily. If you are already filled with answers, if you know so much that you can't pack anything else inside your brain, then you are finished with learning. But if you are able to find space for something new, then you've kept that openness needed for growth. You will continue to find more on the mat, simply by expecting less.

Now I perform and teach yoga practice, not yoga perfection. I come to my mat to acknowledge where I am, and where I'm going. I remember to be grateful that I can even *be* on the mat that day, and that a very busy life did not kept me away.

When you think you know it all, it is the surest way to stop yourself from learning more. When you think you are an expert, yoga is there to prove otherwise. When you think you can't, yoga is there to show you that you already can. I have come to agree with Baron Baptiste, that nothing is more important to me than my own growth. Lucky for us, yoga is there to remind us there is always more.

A Lesson From the Mat

Answers Are Overrated

Ask ten yoga teachers how to do a pose and you will get ten different answers. This often tortures students! In truth, there are probably an infinite number of ways to *do* any pose, and to teach it, depending on what you are looking to accomplish.

Yet yoga is not about the answers. It's about peeling back the mystery of your body, mind and spirit and seeing how everything is connected. That relationship changes over time. As I mature, I have become more comfortable with a lack of knowledge, rather than pretending I know everything. I am happy to discover when I don't know something. Let me study it. Let me ponder it. If I can stay open to new things, open to new ways, if I can keep a beginner's mind, then I think that will make me a better teacher. It will surely keep me a better student for life.

How to Be a Beginner:

- Try not to make assumptions on the mat. Unpack your expectations. Some days are better than others. Be content with your practice that particular day.
- Focus on the important things: your breath, your attitude, how you feel.
- Be grateful there are still certain things you suck at! Hooray for learning.
- Be comfortable with what you don't know.

A Lesson From the Mat

Take Good Notes

In the beginning, everyone loves yoga. Each day brings a huge new triumph on the mat. But after a few months, when the milestones become harder to reach, the student realizes that the work on the mat is actually work, and he often becomes discouraged.

I recognize the signs. It usually sounds like whining, or even quitting. When a student tells me that they feel like they are getting nowhere, this is when I give them a huge hug. "Welcome," I say, "to yoga. Welcome to the rest of your life."

When you see that you know very little and still have a long way to go, it is seeing clearly for the first time. The early joy is like a spell when we fall in love. But eventually, the spell wears off and the relationship will take work and commitment from that time on. The pleasure you felt from getting something new every time you stepped on the mat will now be replaced by the misery of getting nowhere fast.

To keep your practice in perspective, keep a journal of your success. Measure your progress to your desired pose and the steps taken toward your goal. The mind is quick to give up, yet in a journal you will see your improvement, one millimeter at a time.

A Lesson From the Mat

Finding Flexibility

Nothing is more vexing to the tightly bound than flexibility. One thing I have learned on my yoga journey is that anything is possible. Even flexibility for a very tight person is possible. I should know. I could not touch my toes *for five freaking years.* It takes learning and patience. It takes practice. It takes being a good student.

Realize that flexibility is really about strength. To stretch, one must engage the muscle. You cannot have flexibility without strength. To do so, risks a pulled muscle. So the tightly bound have hope.

Get help. Using props such as a block or a strap is not a sign of weakness, it's about going deeper.

Use frustration to gain understanding. Utilize the places where you are stuck to gain new perspective. For example, I was surprised to realize that I could not do the splits because I was tight in the quads, not the hamstrings.

Find ease at the edge. If you can feel at ease in the pose with a steady breath, then you have achieved it no matter what the outer form looks like.

Recognize success. I had gotten so used to not being flexible that I did not realize when I was there. Other yogis began to compliment me on my practice, and I would say, "Oh no, not me." It took me about a year before my brain caught up with my body. Sometimes all we need is to open our eyes and believe in the possibility.

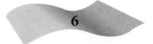

6

Surrender to Grace

There are hundreds of ways to kneel and kiss the ground.

~ Rumi

I come from people who do not surrender.

My family came to America with nothing and made something. These are not people who give up.

My maternal great grandfather was from East Prussia. He moved from Prussia, to Russia, to Germany, to Italy, where he became an artist and a woodcarver. From there, it was Paris, where he met my great grandmother, and then on to London and then America, all to keep his family, then Jewish and Catholic, safe from the horrors of war as anti-Semitism was taking hold. In America, both his children graduated from law school and prospered.

My grandfathers worked hard as well. My maternal grandfather bought passage to America in the cargo hold of a passenger ship with his brother. Once in America, the brothers took turns working days and nights putting each other through law school. My paternal grandfather also came from Europe, arrived with very little, and then worked twelve hours a day in the garment district so my father and his sister could go to college. My father studied so hard, and was so bright, that he went to an Ivy League school at sixteen.

Determination is in my DNA. When you have this much drive and ambition, it is hard to back down. It is hard to surrender, to anything. But this is what I know for sure:

**If you always stay in control,
then you don't allow for the possibility
of "more" to come into your life.**

The simple act of letting something else in, something bigger, something such as surprise and whimsy, could be letting in Grace. Too much control, too much drive and ambition, too much of anything, becomes too little of something else.

In the most trying times of my life, when I have lost a job or lost someone I loved, I thought what I needed was more control, but in fact I needed to be okay with less. These are the times I needed to shut up and listen. Whatever is going to happen, will happen. It takes unbelievable faith to quiet that part of the ego that longs to call the shots. In my case, it just wasn't in my DNA until I got on my mat.

Surrender to Love, But Never Surrender Your Dreams

There are times in life when you do not surrender. You do not lay down without a fight in Nazi Germany. You do not let your teenager skip school because they feel like it. You do not relinquish a dream just because someone else says it's ridiculous. The good fight is always right.

Yet there are also times when you must lay down the sword. The yogi seeks to understand the difference. If you try to be always right, always in control, always on top, you will miss out on the full experience of life. You miss out on the sweetness of love, on what it means to be less, so someone else can be more.

You have closed yourself off from the sweetness of Grace.

When I was young, I had a therapist who told me that to be happy, I must surrender. Now, I am a person who worked hard and although I am mostly a bargain shopper, I've paid full price for everything I had. My innocence about boys was over at twelve. I had been on my own in boarding school and worked in a variety of jobs to make my way. I put myself through graduate school, and have been successful at several careers. And this man was asking me to quit!

"Not quit," he told me, "just put down your guns. If you wave the little white flag, if you say, 'You may be right,' then doors will open for you."

I was thinking, *"What the hell, maybe it is worth a try?"*

It turned out, this man was a genius. And you know what? He *was* right.

Surrender Starts with Thank You

In 2009, I was visiting my family's home on Long Island when I went to a yoga workshop at a studio nearby. I was in a room of superstars: Colleen Saidman and Rodney Yee were there, and so were David Swenson and Beryl Bender Birch.

Now, I wouldn't call my Handstand, *Adho Mukha Vrksasana* glorious. But for my age, it was passable. I could get up. I could stay up. I'm not an ex-gymnast. I'm just a person looking to play the edge in her life by standing on her hands now and then. I mean, playing around in

Handstand is a whole lot better than buying a Porsche or having an affair.

Everything was going fine. We were moving back and forth from Downward Facing Dog, *Adho Mukha Svanasana*, to the front of our mat. Then the time came to spot each other into Handstand. I was first in my group. I checked my foundation, steadied my arms, softened my heart and threw one leg into the air hoping my butt would follow.

Wham. I was up. And I want to be honest here; I'm thinking, *I'm the shit!* I'm in the perfect Handstand. *Whooo hooo, look at me. I'm the bomb.*

Then all of a sudden I heard, a shriek, like a cat with its tail being pulled.

"Oh my Gawd," the woman screamed, "That is a horrible Handstand." Upside down, I am craning my head around to see who she's talking about.

"That is the 'woist' Handstand I have evah seen in my life," she's carrying on like an Evangelist on crack. "Rawwwdney, look at this Handstand. Oh my Gawd."

And I'm looking and looking. I'm craning my neck upside down to see this horrible Handstand. Then in an instant, in a moment of perfect clarity, I realized she was talking about me!

With as much dignity as I could muster, I came down, smoothed my shirt over my mommy belly and put my hair back in place. Then I tried to become invisible while she explained to everyone within fifty miles how horrible my Handstand was. She then jumped upside down to show us what a perfect Handstand should look like.

"That's how you do it," she said.

Let's be clear, "old" Michelle, "un-enlightened" Michelle was very much present.

"*Shut up, bitch,*" is all I wanted to say. "*Shut up because I was Phi Beta Kappa, and I can do a Handstand, and I study with some of the world's greatest teachers, and you've had too much plastic surgery,*" blah, blah, blah.

But this is what happened instead:

The bitch who shut up was me.

It's not easy to shut up and let go of our defenses. The ego puts these walls around us, to protect us, to keep us strong. Yet we must ask ourselves, what are we so afraid of? If I surrender and allow myself to be taken apart, what am I truly giving up? Being right? On the other hand, if I listen, I might learn something new. She might be correct. However, I still have my doubts.

Then—and this is the lesson of surrendering—after the workshop, I walked right up to her and said, "Thank you."

(I know, right? Are you dying? I'm from New York. I could totally have taken this bitch out. But instead, I said *thank you*.)

"What?" she asked, looking down at me.

"You must be a yoga teacher, and so I wanted to thank you for the feedback you gave me about my Handstand. I know I could learn much from you. I only wish I lived in this area where I could study with you regularly." And then I turned around and left her speechless. The strange thing is, a part of me believed it, too.

After dinner that night I dragged my kids down to the beach, and we took snapshots of my Handstand in the surf. I was two parts indignation to one part humility. I must have done about forty Handstands and then studied the photographs. I thought my pose looked pretty good, but if I looked carefully, that woman might have been right. It could be improved.

In fact, everything can be improved. Resistance is the path to stagnation. Being resistant to feedback creates a stagnant life. Being taken apart by this stranger was very hard for me. But what if she was correct? What if I was still just a student and not a teacher? And then the light went on. Shut up, bitch and listen. You might learn something new.

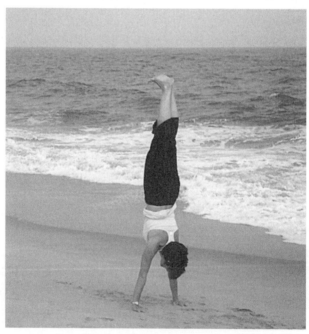

Pose: Handstand, *Adho Mukha Vrksasana*.
After being told my handstand was horrible, I wanted to see for myself.

A Lesson From the Mat

Inversions: The Test of Grace

A Japanese proverb says, "Fall down seven times. Get up eight."

Inversions might be my favorite part of the practice. Not the part I'm best at, but the part where I gain the most clarity.

To practice an inversion is equal parts commanding and surrendering control. To go upside down at fifty years old is either completely insane or courageously trusting in Grace. You need to find calm where there is none. You need to be okay with being very much not okay. It's a lot like life.

As much as I would like to think I have complete control over my life, I just don't. Having control is an illusion, so when we feel we have lost it, we actually see clearly. No matter how good we become at our practice, particularly inversions, there may be some part of the posture we cannot control. And we may fall. Rather, you will fall. Get over it.

If we are not in charge, then who is? To cope with this kind of incomprehensible part of life requires a radical surrender of the ego. To be okay with whatever, that is surrender. To fall and get back up again, that is the test of Grace. All we have to do is accept the gift. Thank you!

A Lesson From the Mat

What It Means to Let Go

There is a fairy tale about a little bug that spent its life clinging to a rock on the side of a stream. It never let go of this rock, for it was terrified of drowning. Then one day, a storm comes along and the rain loosens the bug's grip. It tumbles into the water and quickly finds a way to float. It bounces along until it comes to rest a little ways downstream, where it discovers a colony of bugs just like itself, falls in love, and lives happily ever after.

The fairy tale has a happy ending. In real life, though, there are no guarantees. Yet one thing is for sure: the ego builds up our self-confidence and then in its desire to protect us from harm, it stops our growth. Before we know it, we've been clinging to our little rock for years.

To grow better, to get out of our zip code, to shift into a new realm and to move past our fears into a new self, we have to reposition past the ego just a little bit. This is stepping brilliantly into our fearless heart. Being fearless is not jumping off a cliff without fear. Being fearless is knowing you are afraid and jumping anyway.

If you're not a little afraid, you're stupid. Honor your fear. But have faith that if you let go of the rock you've been clinging to, you might just bounce into a new and wonderful place you were meant to be.

A Lesson From the Mat

Saying "Yes" Is the First Step to Grace

I didn't realize how much I said "No," until I heard myself in the mirror.

When yoga held the mirror to my practice, I realized I was a say "No" kind of person. I had a million reasons to say "No," but very few reasons to say "Yes."

Then my teacher suggested, "Why not say 'Yes'?"

Why not? Or rather, why not start with "Yes" and then move to "Maybe"? I'm from New York, so generally we start with "No," but why not "Yes"? I figured it was worth a try.

A Lesson From the Mat

Thank You Is the New F**k You

This is what yoga has taught me: Becoming enlightened is simple. All you have to do is make *"Thank You"* the new *"F**k You."* I just saved you years of practice and thousands of dollars, not to mention some time in therapy. You are welcome.

Here are several examples of my extreme enlightenment:

- I was practicing yoga and one of the other students commented that they couldn't believe I could still "do it" at my age. *Thank you!*
- My mother-in-law said that she didn't know I worked. Or taught yoga. Or wrote a book. She also told me that for the last fifty years I have been loading the dishwasher wrong. *Thank you!*
- In one year, my father-in-law died, my dog died, my mother was diagnosed with cancer, my husband and I lost jobs, and we were audited by the IRS. So, dear Universe, *thank you!*
- To the yoga studio owner who suggested that I teach "Gentle Yoga for Old People," because I am old and that's what we do, right? *Thank you!*
- And to everyone else who will do me wrong, I appreciate the chance to demonstrate my *uber-yoginess* by saying in advance, *thank you.* Really, I mean it.

PART TWO

Growing Wiser

The Meaning of Alignment

Alignment is wisdom.

If nothing else, as we grow older we should be getting a little wiser. We should know a thing or two by the time it's time.

It is the same in yoga. We seek alignment. We align the muscle and tissue of our bodies so we can straighten our legs and our backs. When our bodies are aligned, they work better, we feel healthier, lighter and more balanced. The practice is also to align ourselves with the world. When we work well with those around us, we feel like we are in the swim of things and not fighting the currents. When our dreams are aligned with reality, they come true. When we are misaligned, everything feels out of place, difficult and forced. We are temporarily at sea.

Alignment is like learning how to play an instrument, but the instrument is you. Learning the "how" of yoga is essential to keep you safe and to help you heal. Sometimes we can become so intrigued with the skill that we can get a little lost in the technicality, becoming Yoga Obsessive Compulsive.

Ultimately, the purpose of yoga is to understand your heart, to perform the highest duty being asked of you. If the path is not yet clear, if you are lost or confused, then the teachings of yoga can lead the way. When practiced with steady and focused attention, alignment becomes an expression of living our lives with clarity and awareness as we seek something more.

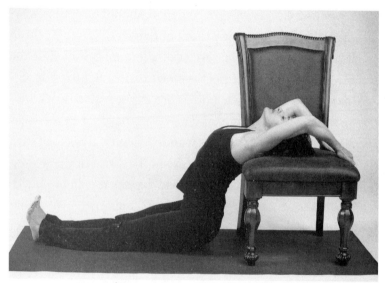

Bridge Pose: *Setu Bandha Sarvangasana,* supported.
The guru within knows when we need help.

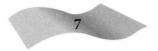

The Teacher Within

You have to grow from the inside out.
None can teach you, none can make you spiritual.
There is no other teacher but your own soul.
~ Swami Vivekananda

We are human, and imperfect is how we roll.

Inherent in our imperfections are the answers to many of our questions. In the stupid things we do, in the mistakes we make, in the enormous challenges we face, we often have the very teachings we seek. Who knew? Actually I did, but it took some time to figure that out.

Like many twenty year olds, after college I didn't know what to do or who I wanted to be. I worked for a year in a law firm, which led me to become a writer. Of course it did! Why go with a surefire career when you could throw it away to be a starving artist? This was right after Watergate, and journalism appeared to be a place where the men looked like Robert Redford and a woman could be taken seriously. The fact that millions of people are now too young to remember that kind of inequality shows the progress we have made. Now that we are enlightened and all this stupid sexist crap is behind us, it is curious to me that yoga studios today actively seek "male energy" on their schedules, which to my way of thinking is no different than it was in the newsrooms and the board-rooms thirty years ago. But I digress.

Back when I first decided I wanted to be a writer and save the world, I enrolled in Columbia University's Graduate School of Journalism, where I spent the next nine months pounding the pavement looking for news and hoping for my big break.

One day a friend invited me to meet a certain famous journalist for dinner. I do not want to say who exactly, but this man changed the course of journalism as well as a bit of world history. He was a crusader for truth and justice. He was even on television! Frankly, I was thrilled to death that I was to meet the greatest living journalist of all time, so I carefully placed the drafts of my stories and my résumé into a brown paper envelope, put on my best skirt and jacket (with bare legs, because in graduate school I could not afford a pair of stockings), and hoping for, I don't know what, perhaps an interview, or a job recommendation, *or a job, please God,* I trotted off like Holly Golightly to a fancy hotel in midtown Manhattan. And there in the lobby was my childhood friend sitting next to my hero, we'll call him "Mr. Superfamous," who was elbow deep into his fourth or fourteenth drink.

We sat and I probably babbled on about how much I admired him, and how he inspired me, and how I wished to be just like him when I grew up (except, possibly sober and without the five o'clock shadow). After yet another drink, the man I worshipped asked if we would like to go upstairs where he had a suite. My friend said sure, and I trotted behind looking for an opportunity to show him my writing.

We entered the suite; my friend went to the bathroom, and the next thing I knew I was pinned under a very sweaty man who badly needed a shave.

I worshipped this man and this is what I got? I thought he was going to be my "teacher," a mentor who would guide me into the depths of the newsroom and help me get a Pulitzer Prize. But instead, I am covered with slobber and all the buttons are torn off my one and only interview jacket.

Don't worry. Absolutely nothing more happened and the only thing wounded was my ego. Once burned, twice shy. Now I would *NEVER* go into a hotel suite with a man I did not know alone. I do not ever walk to my car alone at night. I look both ways, even in the mall. I am the first to call the police when creepy characters hang around the yoga studios waiting for the *yoginis* to emerge.

I am not the small white chick you want to mess with. In this case, my friend came out of the bathroom and Mr. Superfamous rolled off of me. I was not hurt, but I was devastated. And soooo embarrassed. *I thought he would read my stories! I thought he would discover me! I thought he would call CBS and say, "Hire this girl!"* God, how pathetic. Furthermore, I'm not worried about Mr. Superfamous suing me here, because libel is only about what is not true for public figures who have traded their reasonable expectation of privacy for money and fame. I learned that from him.

Because humiliation has no boundaries, the next day my aspiring journalist friends came up to me in school and asked me what Mr. Superfamous was like, since I had mentioned to a few hundred people that I was going to meet him. I told them the truth. I said he did not show up. Because in fact, the legend was somewhere else that evening and instead a lonely, divorced, desperate drunk came in his place.

Who Is the Guru?

Part of getting wiser, part of learning more about who we are and what we want, is figuring out who *exactly* can help us along the way. The guru means one who sheds light, or loosely translated, the one who helps explain all the crap that happens to us, who listens to you whine and still loves you, and who keeps you going even though the odds that you will succeed are like, a billion to one. A guru is a Sherpa; someone who can lead you out of the dark and into the light of your hopes and dreams so you can find your way.

The trick, of course, is to distinguish between your guru and a mistake before you end up pinned on a mattress. Not always easy. It is the same in yoga.

My first yoga teacher who I thought was the "one," passed out in the studio! For two years I thought I was doing "real yoga" with her. And in truth, I was. But in the end, I was interested in going further in my practice and she had gotten off the bus.

Then I moved on to Power Yoga, where I was having the time of my life jumping around on my mat in a heated room. It was fun. It was exhilarating. It was the sweatiest you could get and still be faithful to your husband. Then my body gave me a reality check (*Hellooooo*, you are a middle-aged woman with arthritis so *what the hell* are you doing to yourself?) and one day I could not walk. I knew I had to find another way to practice that was still fun but could also heal my hamstrings. What I didn't realize is that the "something more" could also heal my heart.

I found an alignment style of yoga where the teachers spent so long on one pose that I was pretty sure my freaking arm would fall off. (Although it's never been known to happen, I thought I could be the first to lose a limb practicing yoga.) In addition, the teachers would intertwine the alignment instructions with a little something about how to live a better life. You learn to squeeze your butt with the same desire you might have to be happy, and before you know it, you have a better butt *and you are happy!* Or perhaps you are happy because you have a better butt? Whatever it is, teaching yoga as an offering to being better on and off the mat is pure genius. When yoga is learned from the inside out, what you *feel* is as important a lesson as what you can *do*.

In all of my efforts to find a teacher, a guru or a spiritual guide to greater abundance, I never once considered looking inside *moi!* I thought the experts would always have the answers. But as if to further awaken my totally confused heart, the first words of the invocation I used to sing were to trust yourself, the guru *within*, as well as the one without. Of course! I should have known this long ago. Yet now if given the chance, of all the things I would tell my younger self, I would say stop looking so hard for the teacher without and instead, listen to the teacher within.

Even in youth, we know more than we think we do.
We just lack the confidence to pay attention.

"Don't let the noise of others' opinions drown out your own inner voice," the late Steve Jobs said in a commencement address to Stanford graduates. "And most important, have the courage to follow your heart and intuition."

Learning to listen to the teacher within is growing up; it's getting wiser. It's part of recognizing that we have the answers inside us all along. At the same time, it's helpful to find a guru on the outside who can be a Sherpa to guide us along the way.

Warning: Your Teacher May Be Human

Like lovers, there are so many yoga teachers in the world it is hard to know to whom you should give your heart. Falling in love with your teacher is like falling in love with anyone. There is an element of choosing wisely, and an element of faith. You might pick your teacher because you read about her and chose her specifically, or she might be a total stranger subbing your regular class and you just fall in love. I often wonder do we choose our teachers? Or do they choose us?

Does the Universe choose our teacher?

At times your teacher will shine with life-changing wisdom, and sometimes disappoint you because, *newsflash*, your teacher is human. I have had yoga teachers who I believed were divine beings, and then the following week they came into class drunk. Or one week their theme was inspiring, and the next it was about how their cat threw up. I have had teachers who created brilliant awareness in my body, and then following week, they tweaked my back with an insensitive adjustment. I have had teachers who brought me closer to the Divine, and then later on they said I'd be going straight to Hell because I ate a chicken sandwich. (Actually they may be right, but I'm pretty sure it won't be for the sandwich.)

So if your yoga teacher is human, how will you know if he or she is still right for you despite the obvious human limitations? Here are some clues:

- For some unexplainable reason, you just adore this person. You are drawn to her and you want to cultivate something of her inside yourself.

- Your yoga teacher respects you. We all have an inner teacher: our own wisdom. Your teacher "without" should respect your teacher "within" and the boundaries you set.

- Your needs align. If your yoga teacher only wants to play in Handstand, *Adho Mukha Vrksasana,* and you were hoping to find out why your low back hurts, there is a misalignment.

- Your values align. If you eat meat and this is a HUGE problem for your teacher, a warning light should go off. I also had a teacher who once told me that I could not be a serious yogi because I had children. She suggested that I wait to begin my studies until they went to college. (*I can't make this stuff up.* That's why you found this book on the non-fiction shelf.)

- Ultimately, your teacher will make you feel better, wiser and stronger. You will feel more than, and not less than. Ultimately, just like love, you will know when it is right.

When You and Your Teacher Need to Part Ways

On the other hand, how do you know if your teacher is not your guru?

- If a teacher tells you, "I am the guru, my way is the only way," run as fast as you can. There is no one way to learn, no one way to practice. All paths lead to more awareness. The best yoga is always the one you do.

- If your teacher ignores you. If you fall and are knocked unconscious, and the teacher asks if you could please move outside because your unconsciousness is creating a distraction, you have a problem.

- If you feel unsupported. I had one teacher who told me I did everything wrong. According to her, I held my hands wrong (fingers not spread apart enough); I bent over wrong (arms not outspread); I breathed wrong. *(Listen, bitch, I KNOW how to breathe. I'm 50 and I'm still here.)* Even if you are in a large class, you should feel seen and supported.

- If she spends most of the class demonstrating. Also in this category, if she spends most of the class looking in the mirror, fixing her hair, or doing her nails. *A yoga teacher is there for one reason only: to serve you.*

- If the class does not feel right in your body. Trust yourself about how you feel when you practice and use some common sense about how to avoid injury.

- If your teacher touches you in any way you feel is weird. If you think it's weird, it probably *is* weird.

- If the themes do not shed light on the more meaningful aspects of your life. Themes are not incidental; they are actually an essential ingredient to the understanding of yoga.

I have had all of these happen to me, truly. Now I am to the point where if there is no connection between myself and the teacher, I do not go back for more. My time is precious and my desire to learn is powerful. This is what I know now that I did not know then: my inner guru rules.

A Lesson From the Mat

We Know What Holds Us Back

What do you do when you are stuck in your practice? I believe that a teacher has one part of the solution, and the student has another part.

I once had a student whose tailbone was stuck, which prevented her from doing inversions. At the time she was struggling with Headstand, *Sirsasana*. She flat-out refused to engage the power in her core. In addition, she had pain radiating in her lower body and she was only comfortable when she was overstretching and causing herself more pain. Literally, she sobbed in Child's Pose, *Balasana*, and begged to be taken out.

Because I am generally not in the business of causing people more pain, I looked beyond her practice. Thinking she might have the answer, I asked, "What happened?" (Note to other teachers: If you don't know what to do, just ask your student. They may have the answer.)

I waited, and slowly a light came over her face. She had been raped and sodomized and required multiple surgeries to function. She was also recovering from drug use and bulimia. Instead of using yoga to help build a new foundation, she had been unconsciously turning the practice into another weapon against herself.

I knew that once she made the connection between her pain and her practice, she would be able to make a change. She literally jumped up, scooped her tailbone, engaged her core and went upside down!

As a teacher, I was able to just ask the right question. Yet as a student, she was able to make the powerful connections and be her own best teacher. Her guru was within all along.

A Lesson From the Mat

The Four Stages of Wisdom

Getting wiser is a process. As we mature, we get curious, we ask more questions, we find more answers and possibly we learn a thing or two. Georg Feuerstein describes this cycle with its four distinct stages, in *The Yoga Tradition*.

Stage One: The Student. We start life as a student with the primary duty to become educated. Whether a child or a yogi, the student is eager to learn and willing to grow. In India, a student was assigned to one teacher, studying daily from dawn to dusk.

Stage Two: The Householder. The householder has specific responsibilities. While continuing to study, they are primarily responsible for their home and family. Their *dharma*, or duty, is to take care of the home; study has to take a backseat to everyday life.

Stage Three: The Forest Dweller. The forest dweller's children have grown up and their reward is semi-retirement. The forest dweller has more time to turn to the spiritual path if it does not interfere with his tee time or bridge game.

Stage Four: The Wandering Scholar. The final stage is renunciation, when the elder does not need many worldly goods and is actively seeking a relationship with the Divine instead. This often happens near the end of a person's life cycle (where many of your best clothes may not fit properly anymore, anyway). In Hinduism, the belief is that those whose mind is centered on the Divine, particularly at the moment of death, will either be freed from the cycle of *samsara* (birth, suffering, death and rebirth), or at least have a more favorable rebirth in their next life.

A Lesson From the Mat

Cult or Culture?

Make no mistake. For a yoga believer, I am very skeptical. It comes with the territory of being a New Yorker.

So, it was a surprise, to say the least, when I discovered that my former school of yoga, Anusara, was accused of being a cult! And that the leader was not just human, but deeply flawed. I should have known. I trusted the wrong man before and now I had done it again.

There are many charismatic leaders in yoga and perhaps it is easy to blame them for the obsessed mentality of their followers, but here is the thing: It takes two to tango. As followers, we have the responsibility to think for ourselves. Remember, our guru is inside.

How would you know if you are participating in a positive, life-enhancing yoga experience or drifting into a bizarre situation? You may not know, but here are a few clues:

The Universal Definition of a Cult:

- It has a charismatic leader who is idolized.
- There is devotion to an idea, movement, or school the leader founded.
- The system involves beliefs and rituals.
- The concept is regarded as unorthodox. This "different-ness" creates cohesion among participants and distinguishes the group from any organized religion.
- The perception is that the group can cure disease and bring abundance.

- Money or goods are exchanged. There are dues, payments or donations to the system.
- Those who leave the organization are treated as outcasts.

To be honest, there were some things that I didn't like about my former school, starting with the word, "kula," to describe the community. This word always seemed like "kult-a" to me, and at the very least I recognized it was meant to be exclusive. Yoga, above all else, should be accessible and inclusive of everyone.

In my case, I was a willing participant; I was an "inspired" teacher and nearly "certified." When the founder fell from Grace, many of us were left having spent a small fortune on training that was now worthless. Or was it?

The school was based on a system of alignment that was, for most bodies, truly amazing. I will never regret the training I received, the philosophy I learned, and the skills I have to teach.

I believe that all our teachers, including the ones who abandon us and the ones from whom we separate, were meant to be our teacher. We just may not understand the lesson at the time.

As a yoga junkie, I have had many teachers. Some have broken my heart. Others have healed it.

How will you know if a teacher is right for you? If your teacher brings you joy and healing, if they help you find more on the mat, as well as more out of life, then you know you have found your teacher, or at least one of the many on your journey.

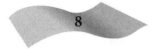

8

Pain Is the Guru

You cannot wage war on the body,
without the violence affecting the mind.
~ Christina Sell

The body never lies. It might whine, but it doesn't lie.

The mind is trickier. You can convince yourself of most anything: I need this new handbag; one more drink won't hurt; and this guy really loves me. Right? But the body gives direct and honest feedback. If you practice out of alignment, it hurts. If you over do, it hurts. If you party all night, it hurts.

"If you are kind to your body, it will respond in the most incredible way," wrote Vanda Scaravelli in her book, *Awakening the Spine.*

Being kind to the body is not always easy.

Like many of us, I have spent a lifetime being most unkind to my body. There were years when I was preoccupied with weight. I tried every kind of diet. (Notice that the word diet comes from "die." Or "weight loss" is about "loss." It's not life affirming at all.) I tried the grapefruit diet until acid reflux almost ripped out my throat. Then there was the pizza diet, which I think was only popular in New York. (The pizza diet is when you tell yourself that every food group is nicely represented on one slice.)

The Atkins diet kept me on the toilet for most of my thirties trying to poop, as I had virtually no fiber in my system. Luckily, I was also toilet training my children, so the three of us would sit for hours having story time on the potty. At least it was quality time.

None of these diets worked in the long term, but it didn't stop me from trying or from hurting my body. Weight is not the only weapon in this war. The real abusers for many of us are the other things we put inside ourselves. I was a child of the Sixties, and like many of us, I inhaled, swallowed, licked and snorted God knows what.

I'm willing to bet that everyone has waged war on their body in one way or another, and woke up in pain one day, even if you won't admit it. Yet as much as pain hurts, it is trying to tell us something. We just need to be better listeners.

Pain Exists for a Reason

Pain can be a guru, but it is up to us to listen. I have come to a point in my life where I am appreciative for the pain and injuries I get because it is a chance to go deeper into my yoga. When I practice with an injury, I am completely awake to the alignment. When I watch my students and friends practice with an injury, I am overwhelmed by the Grace and compassion in their movement. They are filled with sympathy and steadiness.

On the other hand, on the days where I feel healthy and strong, I can mindlessly skim along the surface of the poses, and then, I'll move right out of alignment and slip my sacrum, or pop a rib, or aggravate my shoulder. And it's back to the beginning, one breath, one movement at a time. It's a relief on those days to have no expectations of myself on the mat.

In fact, if it wasn't for the pain in my rear, I would never have been led to greater understanding of alignment in yoga, which changed my practice and my life. So I have learned the hard way:

My body is my muse.

I now listen to my body. But it wasn't always so. Sometimes we don't listen because it is too painful. Or we are just not ready to hear what we already know.

Listen Carefully

There was a time when my body was trying to tell me something and I did not listen. In my first marriage, I went through a period where I could not sleep. I woke up every night at 2:00 A.M. with my heart pounding. I went to the doctor but he found nothing physically wrong. Then he asked me if I was unhappy. I said, "I don't know." Really, *I had no freaking idea.* So I went home and asked my husband, "Are we unhappy?" He left me two months later. I guess one of us was unhappy and one of us was unconscious.

Even in the midst of the happiest times of your life, unhappiness can take hold and not let go. It is like a fog that clings to *every fucking thing in your life.*

I have always been susceptible to depression. You have no idea how hard it is to write that sentence because I have hidden this awful thing for years. I sometimes have depression. I am occasionally depressed. I am sometimes terribly, awfully sad and anxious. It feels good to admit what is real. If I am smiling, I might be lying. If I look cute as a bug, it could be because I am hiding the truth. If you ask me how I feel, and I say, "Great!" just be aware I might be lying like a rug.

When you have depression, it is like a case of mold in the closet or the bathroom. You can scrub and clean and rinse and clean some more and it goes away. Then one day, it's back. I once had some mold in a basement closet and after cleaning it with bleach for six years, I ripped the whole bloody closet out down to the studs. Take that, you stinking depression. Oh, I meant mold. Not as easy to clean up your life.

After my sons were born, I was positively sidelined by depression. Post-partum depression is no joke. After the birth of my children, I was like a zombie spending endless days doing laundry, cooking, cleaning, and wiping little noses and butts. I cried during naptime. I cried at night. I cried just about all the time. My old friend depression came to help with the children, and it settled in for a long stay. If my dearest friend Gwen hadn't also come to help, depression might never have left me in those days.

When Mike saw his wife falling apart, he got me help, lots and lots of help. I had a nanny, a maid, a gardener, a pool boy. (Sounds nicer than it was. In real life, the pool "boy" was about fifty years old, sometimes peed in the bushes, and every month found something that cost $1,000 to fix.) But, like many things we desire, the help turned out to be less helpful and more expensive than we thought. Plus it is really embarrassing to be walking around crying when your house is filled with strangers offering you something to eat so you will feel better. "Enchilada, Missus?"

I thought perhaps that being busy, *really, really busy,* would keep my mind numb. So we let everyone go. I left my job, part time by then, and I became full time "everything" at home. However, though I was busy, I was still not numb enough and the pain seeped through in the quiet moments. I was crying in the car. I was crying in the bathtub. Honest to God, I was crying at the mall, *and who the hell cries at the mall?* So I got help from the new mother's helpers: *Lexapro, Zoloft, Wellbutrin.* It's all the same. I spent five years on the stuff, and while I don't regret it, it didn't make me happy either. It just made me numb. I was numb so I could cope.

But coping isn't living. Coping isn't feeling. Coping is some place between life and death. Then one day, after about seven years of coping, I decided that enough was enough. If depression was bad, then not having it was worse. When I was on the "mood enhancers," I was not enhanced. I could not taste my food. I could not feel my husband's touch (or even my own!); I could not enjoy my children's love. I didn't suffer, but I also didn't have pleasure. I was not "more." I was less.

So I did what I've always done when I felt lost: I went home to Mom. I went off the pills one day, and believe me it was bad, with lots of crying and vomiting. For two weeks I lay on her couch with migraines, nausea and weakness as I adjusted to life without meds. Note to all my friends who have been there: you should probably do this gradually, especially if you've been on these pills for some time. That is what the doctors recommend.

One week into my self-prescribed detox, I crawled off the couch and decided to go for a walk. At the time Mom lived in a college town in Florida. I wandered among the damp green foliage and soggy flowers. (It is always soggy in Florida.) Pretty soon I found myself in a city memorial filled with statues of heroes from America's wars. I was surrounded by huge iron warriors, men with guns on horseback, riding tanks and submarines, and I'm wondering: *How did I get here?*

I used to be the bravest person I knew, and now, I was a nauseous, nervous wreck. I felt so weak and out of control. I started to cry. So right there in the Garden of Military Statues surrounded by these giant iron men, I took Child's Pose, *Balasana.* I huddled into my breath. I did the only rational thing I could think of: I prayed. I asked God to please help me feel better so I could be a good mom again. I wanted to live again, and live fully. After breathing and praying, for I don't know how long, I felt well enough to try a few Sun Salutations, *Surya Namaskars.* Seriously, I stayed in that garden for an hour practicing *Virabhadrasana,* Warrior poses until I felt calm enough to face my own battles at home.

Teacher, Heal Thyself

The best advice I ever received was if you are in pain, find a teacher who has had the same kind of injury, because a teacher who has healed themselves can then heal you.

When I returned home detoxed and clear-headed, I went looking for a teacher to heal me. I was looking for a yoga teacher who was a former executive who left a job she was great at, to be a mom (which she's not so great at), who has had a shoulder, hamstring, wrist, elbow, upper, mid- and lower-back, knee and everything-in-between injury, who used to take too many pills, and who now occasionally takes too many drinks, because I want to live a better life.

Oh, one more thing. I want to forgive all the people who did shit to me because everyone says it will make me happy. *Hell yes.* I do not know for sure why we suffer, but I do know this:

Pain is a great teacher.

Pain is the four-alarm fire going off in your body to let you know, *"Helllooooooooo, there is a problem here. You might want to slow down and listen."* Pain is the mystery of concealment, where we do not know what is wrong, but if it's loud enough and gets our attention, perhaps we'll listen. And then from pain, from the desire to understand, comes the simplicity of revelation. This makes us wiser.

I was lucky to have found not one, but many great teachers to help guide me through this time. While workshops and retreats were amazing restoratives, there is nothing better than finding a local teacher to learn from on a weekly basis. Sometimes my pain and anxiety could not wait until the March weekend getaway; I had to practice right then. And finally, I decided to step up and be a better teacher for all those other recovering corporate executives with small children and anxiety who were seeking some relief and a bit of humor in the situation. Come to me; we'll laugh and practice yoga through the tears.

When we are young, we can get away with all kinds of bad behavior done to ourselves. We bounce back from all-nighters and a poor diet, from broken hearts and bad choices. We can drink and drug and then wake up and do it again until one day we feel terrible and it doesn't get better. As we age, it's harder to recover. Poor alignment in our practice can put us in traction. A poor diet leaves us feeling weak.

So the question becomes, how do you want to live? Do you want to cope, or live out loud? Do you want less, or do you want more?

Experience has taught me to take care of my body because it's the only one I've got.

I hope to be practicing yoga, and skiing, and hiking for a long time.

I hope to be fully present, fully alive for at least fifty more years.

I hope to be there for my children and their children for many years.

I want to be the skiing grandma who can also stand on her head. For me, that is living more meaningfully for as long as I am here.

A Lesson From the Mat

Practice Peace—*Ahimsa*

Learning to be kind to ourselves is really at the heart of our yoga practice. It goes to the heart of the Sanskrit word *ahimsa*, to do no harm. We start with ourselves.

When we practice yoga, each pose becomes an offering to the highest. If you can achieve new depth even for one or two seconds, the experience is pure bliss, *ananda*. It is a glimpse into our greatness. But you cannot experience bliss if you are engaged in a war on any level.

Working through pain, working against pain, ignoring pain, are wars against the body. The pain exists to get your attention. Of course, we love the poses, but we have to love our body first. Loving your body *is loving you*.

Honor thy body; it is the only one you get. If there are days when your balance is off, then hold onto a wall or a chair. If there are days when you do not feel well enough to go upside down, then don't go upside down. If there are days when your breath is short and shallow, then by all means focus on nothing more than inhaling and exhaling in a comfortable seated position.

In practice, if I am at the edge of my abilities, I wait. There is no hurry. There is always tomorrow. Every pause becomes a chance to observe and learn. While growing older has given me many gifts, the greatest is compassion, not only for others but also for myself. I've learned that sometimes backing off a posture is love. Sometimes going deeper is love. Knowing the difference is wisdom.

A Lesson From the Mat

You Are What You Eat and Drink, Part One

Certain schools of yoga require vegetarianism as a form of *ahimsa*—to do no harm, choosing not to support the killing of animals. However, in my opinion, there is no "right" answer to the challenge of how to eat. You have to do what is appropriate for you, keeping in mind what is right for your family and for the world.

Making everyone else "pay" for your choice of diet and principles isn't ideal either. When I first became a yogi, I tried to keep my house closer to a vegetarian, low fat diet because it was healthy and kind to animals. Then my son broke his arm, and then broke it again. One mother asked me if I felt guilty for feeding him a low-fat diet. I didn't feed him a completely low-fat diet, but I still felt guilty because perhaps there were a few too many "meatless Mondays" in the average week for a growing boy. Guilt is like nectar for moms.

Truthfully, I don't like diets and cleanses that are not nourishing to the body. The ideal weight is the one where you feel strong and healthy, not when you are stumbling around faint from lack of food. My practice tells me what I need to know more than the scale. If I gain a few pounds and cannot haul my *"ass-ana"* into a Handstand, I will eat more fruits and vegetables until I am back to where I can float in the air. (Although those tight yoga pants tell me a good deal as well.)

In my opinion, the yogic way is not one path or the other. The yogic way is to be conscious and aware, eating in a way that causes the least amount of harm and the greatest amount of good, for oneself and for all other beings.

A Lesson From the Mat

You Are What You Eat and Drink, Part Two

A few things to consider that you may not have considered or that you may have considered to be utter nonsense. But here they are anyway:

Practice peace in your diet. When you ingest a food, you may also ingest its *karma*. The former boxing champion Mike Tyson recently disclosed that he is a vegetarian because he does not want to ingest any more anger. There is the possibility that when you eat an animal, you ingest not just the protein, but also the animal's *karma* as well. If the animal is factory-farmed and stressed, depressed, diseased, scared or angry, those hormones become a part of you. I try to choose animal products from farms that give the animals a good, healthy life, and then one bad day.

Consider the source of the egg. Several years ago McDonald's announced they were going to invest in chicken farms to increase the quality of their eggs. Come on, if McDonald's is concerned about the eggs they use, we ought to be in a panic. Look for the egg with the darkest richest yolk, from the freest bird that eats the best food and lives the closest to you that you can afford.

Make conscious choices. If you drink, be aware that you may not be able to balance the next day. If you spend the night around smoke, your breath will probably be constricted the next day. If you want to practice strong, then make appropriate decisions.

Lower your carbon footprint. You can support your local economy by choosing foods that are grown close to home. The supermarket in my neighborhood labels the Colorado produce. Farmer's markets are also ideal. Buying a berry from another continent in the middle of winter is hard on the planet.

Ponder your protein source. Red meat is the most carbon-intensive food, and dairy is right up there. However, chicken, fish, and eggs are less carbon intensive to produce than fruits and vegetables. It's just another way to consider causing no harm to the planet.

Ahimsa **first.** Some of my favorite vegetarians have a bite of bacon every now and then. *Ahimsa*, to do no harm, also means non-judgment. It is the first of the *Yamas*, or the ethics of behavior in the *Yoga Sutras*. Have compassion first, and then try non-judgment.

Look at the big picture. You don't have to become a vegan and drive a Prius to make a difference for our planet. You can take baby steps. One meatless meal; choosing a paper bag over a plastic bag; buying re-useable glass water bottles instead of plastic throw-aways; walking instead of driving to get a carton of milk or pick up your kids in the neighborhood—these little steps add up over time. No effort is wasted. It all helps in the end.

A Lesson From the Mat

Concealment and Revelation

This much I know for sure: The answers are revealed to us only when we are ready to understand them. A cycle of learning has to happen. Although frustrating at times but necessary, pain and sickness are examples of concealment. Sometimes we don't know why, but if our pain is bad enough, we'll seek the answers.

In the Hindu depiction of Dancing Shiva, *Nataraja*, the God of Destruction has one foot on the demon dwarf Apasmara's head. He could easily crush this small being, but Shiva keeps him around instead. Why? Because the dwarf is a symbol of our limited self, of our ignorance, concealed from the truth and obscured from enlightenment. Shiva honors the time of concealment as a necessary prelude to enlightenment. We would not seek the answers if we had them. That is just the way we roll.

Likewise, in the epic poem the *Bhagavad Gita*, the warrior Arjuna asks Lord Krishna to tell him what to do. It takes Krishna eighteen long chapters to get to the point, because until then, Arjuna is not ready to hear the truth. Later in the story, Arjuna asks to see the Universe, kept inside of Krishna's mouth. Krishna obliges and shows him everything, the whole enchilada, but Arjuna becomes sickened by the sight. "Have mercy," he said to Krishna. It was too much at once.

Concealment is frustrating. Revelation can be overwhelming. Learning to listen and wait for the answer is the path to greater wisdom.

9

Desire Takes You Shopping

It's not the having, it's the getting.
~ Elizabeth Taylor

I shop, therefore I am.

I am my grandmother's daughter. She raised me in the hallowed halls of Saks Fifth Avenue and Lord & Taylor. Her idea of a perfect day always began with a sale and a pair of shoes that matched her bag. At the end of his days, my husband would like his ashes to be spread across Flathead Lake in Montana where he grew up swimming, fishing, hunting and waterskiing. Me, I'm thinking Bloomingdales.

My first yoga training was of the more traditional sort. There it was taught that desire was bad, bad, bad. You are a naughty doggy for wanting more.

"So much of yoga has become about the perfect pants and not about our spirit," said my teacher, with some disgust.

News flash: If I ever find a pair of yoga pants that hides my middle and lifts my rear that has long since descended into the back of my knees, I am buying six pairs. No, make it sixty. But in an effort to fit in, I tried to look "spiritual" in baggy pants with sweat stains. Actually, I have done a pretty good job.

The Buddhist view is that the root of mankind's trouble is desire. We desire, therefore we suffer. Or, we desire, therefore we suck as enlightened beings. Either you get what you want or you don't get what you want, but whichever way, you're screwed. The solution is to end your desire by cutting yourself off completely from the manifest world. You know, go to the top of a mountain where there are no showers or health spas and meditate for the rest of your life. Easier said than done.

Eve could have anything, but the one thing she was told she could not eat brought down paradise. Lord Shiva meditated for ninety-nine years in a cave so he would not want anything worldly, but most of all so he would not want his beautiful wife, Parvati. But despite his effort, his desire for Parvati brought him back into the world. If the greatest warrior of all time could not rid himself of desire, then how will it go for us mortals?

The Tantric philosophy is different from classical schools of yoga. Tantric theory says that life is not a problem to be solved, but a contradiction to be embraced. Therefore, if we deeply desire something, then perhaps we should get it.

You are not a terrible yogi for having desires, even if what you want is a new handbag.

It is desire that helps us live a more fulfilled life. Desire alerts us to what we want. It's like a two-page ad in the Sunday paper; our fulfillment wakes us up. If what we want is a better job, then we should go get it. If we want better health for our family, then we should provide better food. If we want a new pair of boots, then we should earn a little more *moolah* to make it happen.

However, if you want something so bad that it becomes a single-minded obsession, then that also inhibits your success. If you practice yoga five hours a day and do not take care of your family, it becomes a problem (speaking from experience). Same with spending the entire day at the mall looking for that one thing you really, really want, that you may not be able to afford (hmmm, also speaking from experience). Yet if you can find a way to desire something, but not want it so much that it ruins your life, if you can desire it so you can manifest it, but also live without it, then *voilá*, the Universe delivers. It's crazy, but true.

Universe, take me shopping!

The Pursuit of Happiness

My own battle with desire these days is not so much about the perfect shoes or the ultimate bag; certain poses are my fixation instead. My husband says that yoga is saving him all kinds of money at the mall, even though I still don't get dinner on the table.

At first, all I wanted was to do the splits, *Hanumanasana*. I struggled with this pose for years. Forty-five years to be exact. Although there are many yoga teachers who are naturally flexible, I am not one of them.

My journey to *Hanumanasana* culminated in a humiliating moment with my teacher, Amy Ippoliti. I was humbly perched like a rag doll on blocks: blocks under my hands, blocks under my thighs and blocks under my *"ass-ana"* as I gingerly lowered myself down into something vaguely looking like the splits.

"Oh fucking hell," I screamed. (I know, this is not what you want to hear from your yoga teacher. We are supposed to be serene, and even-tempered, like the Mona-you-know-what-Lisa.)

My yoga buddy Celia was also suffering and struggling with the pose on the mat next to me. But instead of swearing, she would breathe. Well, I'm breathing like a freight train and it's not working. But here's Celia doing the tranquil yogi thing and looking almost perky. She was even smiling! Before this yoga Immersion, Celia had rarely if ever, heard the "F" word in her life, so I'm proud to say I've given her a whole new education.

If desire had an ultimate mission, it would be to alert us to reality. By noticing what we want versus what we have, we become more aware. By noticing that my hamstrings were as supple as a steel cable, I was awakened to what I really wanted: better flexibility.

You have to wake up from the coma of modern-day life, to go for what you really want.

Notice If You Have Arrived

Desire and discontent keep us off balance. They keep us humble. From that place, we can strive for more in our lives. Living in that in-between place, between what you want and what you have, is uncomfortable at best and miserable at worst.

But becoming comfortable in the uncomfortable, or stepping into the natural flow of life without struggle, is finding balance in an off-balance way. To me, that is one meaning of yoga. And above all other emotions, desire is at the heart of my practice.

So, painfully aware of my desire to be flexible, I set off to change things. I started with a steady approach to the Monkey Pose. I practiced at least five times a week. I kept a journal and measured on a weekly basis the actual distance I was from the ground. And one millimeter at a time, I inched toward a full *Hanumanasana*.

"Never, never, never give up," said Winston Churchill. I would have said it first, but Churchill beat me to it.

It took me five years, but I got the pose. I did not even realize it at first, but a teacher pointed it out to me. I was so used to the chasing, to the desiring and the hopelessness that I had not realized I had arrived. I was in a room with a *Dharma Mittra* teacher in Colorado, when he complimented every student on their effort in the posture, except me. Of course!

"Excuse me," I said, trying to breathe (and actually not swear in public) as I was tentatively lowering myself down, "but I have been working on this pose for it seems like my entire life. Can you tell please me when am I going to get it?"

"Are you kidding me?" he said. "You already have it."

I'm thinking, *This is a load of yoga bullshit*, but to humor him, I look down, and I realize, wow, maybe I do have something of a Hanuman pose? It's not a good-looking Hanuman.

It's certainly not a perfectly aligned Hanuman. But perhaps, it's *my Hanumanasana*. And just like that:

**Desire's secret mission was completed:
I realized I had arrived.**

I wondered, what if we all already had what we were looking for, but failed to see it? What if the Universe was taking us shopping for something we had the whole time?

By the way, I thought for sure that if I ever got *Hanumanasana*, I would never, ever, desire another thing on the mat. I would be so happy and content. I would be in this thing called *samadhi*, the ultimate peace. But guess what? I really want to do a press-up Handstand, *Adho Mukha Vrksasana*. And I know if I get there, I'll be satisfied. Really, that's all I'll ever want. Universe, are you listening?

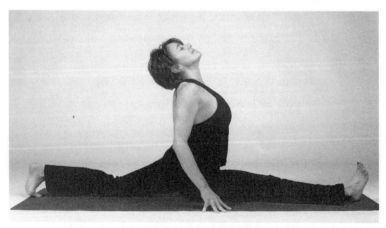

Pose: *Hanumanasana,* Splits.
I wanted this pose for so long, I didn't realize when I had it.

A Lesson From the Mat

The *Ramayana*

The *Ramayana* was one of the earliest stories of desire. Before Adam and Eve, before Romeo and Juliet, before Michelle and the Mall, there was Rama and Sita.

Rama was an incarnation of Lord Vishnu, the most beloved and wisest of the Gods. Sita was an incarnation of Lakshmi, the most beautiful of all Goddesses. Rama and Sita were the Homecoming King and Queen of the Hindu world.

Yet for complicated reasons, they were banished to the forest. One day while walking in the woods, Sita was stolen by Ravana, the king of the neighboring island of Sri Lanka. She shed her jewels little by little as she was being abducted to leave a trail for her husband, Rama to follow. While possession is nine-tenths of the law, it cannot claim the heart. Sita loved only Rama.

Rama's nature was that of peacekeeper and ruler; he was not a warrior. So he enlisted the help of the glorious monkey God, Hanuman to rescue Sita. Hanuman followed the trail of jewels, then jumped across the ocean (in the yoga pose resembling the splits) to save Sita. But she was not impressed, chiding Hanuman, "Excuse me? Where's my man?" Sita refused to be rescued until Rama got off his throne to come for her himself. So long story short, Rama waged a war and won her back.

I would like to tell you that one of the oldest stories of love and desire had a happy ending, but in truth, not so much. Sita had to go through a trial by fire to prove her purity after the years spent with Ravana waiting for Rama to come get her. (I prefer the "don't ask, don't tell" approach.) She survived, but unfortunately, doubts about her virtue lingered. Both Rama and Sita suffer in the end.

I really don't know what this means about desire, except that sometimes we may not know when we already have it pretty good.

A Lesson From the Mat

Think Before You Buy—Anything

Years ago yoga used to be about finding a bit of mental clarity in meditation, which required a mat and perhaps a cushion. Today, however, yoga is a multi-billion dollar industry. There are major international corporations in the yoga business, with festivals, conferences, retreats, videos, accessories, and mainly, clothing.

When I first started to practice, especially in the heated rooms, I used to roll out of bed and go to my class in my pajamas. I figured if I was going to get sweaty and ruin my hair, why bother looking nice? Then I learned that when you practice yoga, you should show up lovely, as a gift to the Divine, because your practice is an offering to the Highest. As a gift, who wants a dirty girl in pajamas?

I interpreted this as a need to shop. (Yoga just kept getting better and better!) As I hit the stores, and more recently online, I discovered there are many issues that divide the yoga community about their yoga pants.

Should yogis:
- Wear clothes that are not organic and therefore harm the environment?
- Support companies that use off-shore manufacturing and perhaps unfair labor?

Of all the issues swirling around yoga marketing, certain upscale retailers are causing divisiveness. One retailer's yoga pants are expensive, made overseas, with mostly non-organic materials, and probably by enslaved and disabled infants working 24-hours a day. At this time, clothes for larger sizes and those for the older yogi (who may want to retain a sense of dignity when going upside down) are difficult to obtain.

The bottom line is you have to feel good about what you buy. You have to feel good in what you wear. Yoga is a practice to better oneself and the world, and you can't do this if you are supporting companies that cause harm.

However, I also like to look cute. It is not "more yogic" to show up on your mat in old gym clothes. It is not "less yogic" to wear a matching outfit. Everyone has to do what is right for him or her. Yet I do know this: There are a whole lot of people who say they practice non-judgment, who pass a whole lot of judgment about what people wear on the mat.

A Lesson From the Mat

What I Desire Most

If desire manifests reality, then this is my shopping list:
- A good night's sleep.
- Happy and healthy children. (And please God let them be successful so they move out of the house someday, but not too far away.)
- Time to make a dinner party and invite my five best friends.
- Five best friends to invite to a dinner party.
- To be a better friend, wife and mother, yet not necessarily in that order.
- *Adho Mukha Vrksasana*, Handstand; *Kapotasana*, King Pigeon Pose; *Dhanurasana*, Full Bow Pose with Arms Overhead; *Parsva Kukkutasana*, Twisted Rooster; blah, blah, blah.
- To not give a shit about the things I shouldn't give a shit about.
- To live fully.
- To love completely.
- To be happy, most of the time.

10

Cancer Sucks

To conquer fear is the beginning of wisdom.
~ Bertrand Russell

The light was blinking red on the answering machine.

It was Sunday night and I had an odd feeling. The soon-to-be ex and I had just returned from visiting his daughter from the first of his serial marriages. It was a long road trip and we were tired from the drive, tired from trying to be careful with each other, gingerly picking our way through a landscape littered with the remnants of a thousand disappointments. Unknown to us, the final landmine in our short marriage was about to go off.

I pressed the button and heard my doctor's voice. For a second I wondered, why would my doctor be calling me on the weekend?

We had been married about a year at this point, and I'm thinking, let's have a baby. *Right?* I'm asleep in this marriage, worrying about food mixers and blenders, and now I want a baby. I can't get dinner on the table, but I want a baby. We can barely pay the rent, but I want a baby. My husband is banging the former assistant city editor's wife, but I want a baby.

I spent a lifetime worrying about getting pregnant, and now I couldn't. It wasn't just that I was older, because truly the only women who have no trouble getting pregnant whatsoever are teenagers. But now, my period had stopped. (God works in mysterious ways.) At first, I'm jumping up and down and rushing out to buy those home-testing kits. But the strips keep saying negative. So I buy more kits and try harder to aim my pee at the ridiculously tiny little square on the end of the stick. And still, no positive, no period and no baby. So I went to the doctor.

The fertility odyssey sets sail slowly. It took me a few months of working eighty hours a week as a journalist before I realized that perhaps I was missing something. In fact, I hadn't had a period in quite awhile. Then you rationalize things so it's not so scary. Maybe I'm anemic? Maybe I need more sleep? (Sorry to say, "Maybe I need a new husband," didn't come to mind.)

And then the answer comes in a blinking red light on a Sunday night.

Cancer.

Ironically, or perhaps as part of the Universe's master plan, my cancer had nothing to do with the missing period. But if not for the missing period (due to a hormone imbalance that led to the infertility), I wouldn't have seen a doctor. And if I hadn't seen a doctor, the silent enemy would have been allowed to grow deeper inside me, taking over new territory and recruiting new cells until the fight was over before I might have known I was in a battle in the first place.

Cancer may take months or years to develop, but when the diagnosis comes, everything happens very fast. The voice on the machine said I had an appointment Monday morning with an oncologist. I was sure this had to be a mistake. I was only twenty-nine years old. I ate my fruits and vegetables. I tried to be a good person and I even helped old ladies cross the street. This should not be happening to me.

**Let me tell you about fear.
It is real, and it is always present.**

Fear

When you cannot see the enemy, it is the worst. If you have ever lost anything that truly mattered, like your freedom, or your health, or someone you loved, then you know there is a lot in the world that can cause us harm.

The reality is that fear is always with us. It creeps about in the corners of our existence. You can try and carry a big sword, cutting away at the things you think might bring you harm. But in fact, you'll cut away the good *and* the bad. The enemy is sneaky; it hides itself deep down in your gut.

So how do we live with such a clever adversary? Very carefully.

Here is what I learned about fear that Sunday night. Despite spending the night crying, with my head in the toilet vomiting, despite shivering under the covers, despite holding my soon-to-be ex's hand and trying to believe his promises that we would get through this together, despite all the late night TV I watched when I could not sleep, the morning came right on schedule. Yup. Sun came up. No matter how afraid you are, the world keeps right on going.

When I arrived at the oncologist's office, she took a biopsy of my cervix (which is code for causing the most pain I have ever felt except for childbirth) and announced she thought from the looks of things, the cancer may have spread to my uterus. Just like that, it was goodbye baby. Goodbye hopes and dreams. Goodbye to the girl who was living in La La Land. Hello to the woman who just woke up and realized she would be lucky to live at all. A hysterectomy was scheduled for the next week.

So, you know that is not how the story ended. You know this because on the book jacket it says I have kids—two in fact. And if you read Chapter 2, you know I had those boys the old fashioned way—with morphine.

But this is the thing about fear:

Fear is about the unknown.

At the time, I did not know there was going to be a happy ending when I went under the knife. With my best friend by my side (I know, right? *Where's the ex-husband?*), I had to sign a waiver saying I understood my doctor would keep removing cells until she had a clean sample, and if necessary, that would mean uterus, ovaries, tubes and all. I understood this was possibly the end of my hopes for a family. Yet the choice was easy. I wanted to live.

When I woke up there was good news: I still had my uterus. The doctor said that after chemotherapy, I would probably be able to have a child in the future.

A child. The future. I clung to her words with feverish intensity. A child. The future.

Yoga Confronts Your Fears

B.K.S. Iyengar said that the reason he practiced Headstand, *Sirsasana,* everyday well into his nineties is to confront fear. I get that. Being courageous, having a fearless heart, isn't about going forward when you have nothing to fear. *It's about going forward when you have everything to fear, and you continue anyway.* It's about remembering that the sun will come up the next day, and the next, and the next. You go ahead partly because you have no other choice, and partly because you choose to.

For some reason, as I get older, I get more afraid. Rape, cancer, and divorce: I hit the trifecta before I was thirty years old. Statistically, the future should be great! Yet if I am to live with a fearless heart, then I must learn to trust that the future is bright.

What makes us believe that even if we survived the past, we won't be able to survive the future?

We are quick to accept as true that we will collapse when we need to be strong. What if, and this might be crazy, insane, radical thinking—what if the qualities in us that helped us endure to this point, what if those same qualities are enough to keep us going full throttle to handle whatever the world brings us in the future? What if? Could you believe in it enough to make it come true?

The real reason I come to my yoga mat almost every day, isn't just to improve my practice, or ease an aching muscle, or even to find peace. The real reason is to face my fears and to embrace my strength.

As we get older, our worries can get the best of us. My grandmother would watch CNN and call me every time she saw a tornado in the Midwest terrified it would sweep me up in its wake. I would reassure her the tornado is not near Denver, but it did little to calm her down.

Fear can take us over, or we can stand our ground. I wage the battle on my mat with a wobbly inversion, or perhaps a claustrophobic forward fold, or a huge yawning backbend. All deep poses scare the shit out of me. Yet, I go specifically where I am afraid to go, and I feel a little stronger afterward. Despite my fear, I keep my heart lifted and bright and soft. This is my way of saying, *I'm still here! That's right cancer and divorce and all the other stuff I endure.* I'm still here. I'm still standing in the light, and I'm getting better, wiser and stronger.

Once, I made the mistake of feeling so strong that I told the Universe to bring it on, and we were greeted with an audit by the IRS the following week. So, I'm not recommending being badass about it. Just optimistic.

In addition, I choose my teachers carefully. If you are looking to go somewhere scary, like inside, having the right yoga teacher helps. You should feel just a little braver afterward. Your teacher should make you feel like you are in this together, and they will stay by you, no matter what.

Life Goes On

The cancer story never ends; it only goes into remission, like an intermission in a play. The second act waits and waits and waits for you. Cancer hangs around forever. You get to tell every doctor, every lover, even the beauty spa wants to know if you've had cancer before they give you a facial. And if you forget, a bad pap smear will remind you thirty years later. But while cancer was just beginning its relationship with me, it turned out to be the end of my relationship with the ex. One year into our marriage, we had stepped onto a landmine that set a blast too big to escape.

Chemotherapy left me temporarily unable to have sex and that was that. He left four months later for the wife of another man.

Of the terrible things I have done in my life, and I have done plenty, I regret to this day one thing: When my ex left with the former assistant city editor's wife, a pudgy little blonde who, on a good day, resembled Miss Piggy, *I did not tell her.* My ex was probably only the second man who ever told her she was beautiful, and she grabbed at the brass ring of happiness without looking twice. She certainly did not look back at me, the road kill of their love affair. She did not think twice about the woman who was sick and without family in Ohio, without a job or even a home because we were planning on moving together to the other side of the country. I did not know when I gave my notice at work and sold everything that she was in the passenger seat, not me. No, she did not think about me. But this was my sin: I did not consider her either.

At the time, I did not mention to her that I had cancer, and that the disease that caused this thing could potentially be transmitted to her. You see, cervical cancer is caused by a virus that is spread primarily through sex. There is a stigma attached to it, but the way I see it, is if you are going to bake bread, then you will probably get covered in flour. And I had baked some bread in my day. So had my ex. I might be wide-awake and fully alive with the pain of knowing. But she was unaware, sleepwalking into a new marriage with a potential time bomb silently ticking deep inside her. My sin was that I did not consider her at all.

I figured I was 29, divorced, alone. I was in chemotherapy and a lot of pain. I was worried about my hair and my health, not to mention my life. I had no home, no job, and was pretty much, at the bottom. And she was on her honeymoon. *Que sera sera. Right? Que fucking sera.* Yet, I still regret that decision.

A Lesson From the Mat

We're in This Together

When you come to the mat, relax. Everyone is afraid. This is what I know for sure having been on my mat for nearly twelve years, and teaching for almost half as long. Everyone is afraid. Take comfort in knowing that you are not alone. The fact that you even went into a yoga studio, that you will be seen in some kind of spandex, that your hair is not done and your pedicure may be chipped, and you will probably fail at some crazy ass pose—in front of everyone—is proof that you are way ahead of the game.

Fear is the ego holding on to what it has. It's like a toddler who walks around saying, "Mine, mine, mine," annoying the hell out of everyone else. When the ego feels threatened, perhaps because we are growing older and weaker, it tries to protect what it has. The ego clings to what it knows, and it does not like the unknown.

Yoga is lovely as a group effort. Together we can face our fears on the mat. In yoga, we are here to support and love each other. You find that with encouragement, you can do incredible things. The desire for freedom can outweigh fear. And with this many people pulling for you, you can go forward with more confidence and let your inner badass burn bright.

A Lesson From the Mat

Become Skilled with the Unknown

I laugh at those who say, "There's nothing to be afraid of." Baloney. Fiddle Faddle. Hogwash. If you have lived to the ripe old age of thirty, or forty, or ninety, you know, there is plenty to be afraid of. Even the twenty year olds today face the worse job market in recent history. For sure, we have lived through some terrible things. That is the human experience!

So why pretend you are something you are not? A former gymnast may be able to jump into a Handstand in the middle of the room, but what about the rest of us? If you are a middle-aged scaredy cat who's never been upside down in your life, it might be a good idea to learn how to do it first. Just sayin'.

These days I see a lot of yoga instructors teach the inversions as a means to confront your fears. Jump in and you will be saved. *Praise the Lord.* In actuality, I jumped up into my first Handstand, fell over backwards, and knocked myself unconscious. Wow, I am *so* not over my fear. Inversions do help us to master fear; however they also have the potential to be change agents and teach about our practice. If you can fill the back of your waist standing up, the next test is to do it upside down. If you can rotate your legs correctly while walking, try doing it in the air, and so on. Inversions point out to us the places in our practice where we need to hone our skills. I consider the inversions as a way to become more skilled with the unknown, to have respect for the things we fear, and to help us live peacefully with so much uncertainty in life. They are not just about mastering fear. They are about mastering life.

You will know when you are ready to take an inversion into the middle of a room. Be patient. It may be in a few months, it may be in a few years. It may be on certain days and not others. But I can't stress this enough: being ready is not about just being unafraid. It's about being skilled, and trusting that your skills will prevail over your fears and plunging ahead anyway. That's living with a fearless, not a foolish, heart.

A Lesson From the Mat

Embrace Your Suckiness

You will fall. You will fail. And you will survive. How do I know this? Because I already have failed at something and survived.

Once I was studying with my teacher in Denver working on kicking up to Handstand in the middle of the room. I was at the point where I could maintain my balance, but I could not willingly, consciously put myself in this kind of danger.

"What are you afraid of?" he asked me.

"I am afraid I'll fall."

"You will fall," he said. "You absolutely will fall."

"Oh, that's reassuring," I said.

"Yes, it is," he said. "You will fall, but you will be alright. You will get back up, and you will be better at it the next time. I promise."

I have fallen many times. I fell in Crow, *Bakasana*, and nearly broke my nose. I fell in Handstand, *Adho Mukha Vrksasana* and knocked myself unconscious. I fell in Revolved Crescent Lunge, *Parivrtta Anjaneyasana* and took out an entire row of a room including a very sweet, very old woman who didn't weigh more than a small bird. I fell in Half Moon Pose, *Ardha Chandrasana*; Forearm Stand, *Pincha Mayurasana*; and Headstand, *Sirsasana*, to name a few. And I'm still here.

At the end of the day, I'm not afraid to suck at yoga, and I feel a little less afraid just because I tried. We could stay in a beginner class for the rest of our lives, but what would be the fun in never falling? After you fall, you should stand taller simply for having tried.

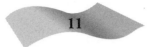

Analysis Paralysis

Many people try to think their way into an asana,
but you must instead feel your way into it
through love and devotion.
~ B.K.S. Iyengar

"Yoga is 99% practice and 1% theory," said Sri K. Patabhi Jois.

I have confused that ratio most of my life, trying to think my way through all kinds of situations. There are some things, however, you cannot think your way through. You have to *feel* your way instead.

I am more comfortable with the thinking rather than the feeling. However, there are times in life when things happen that wake you up to the fact that you are not in charge.

The Vacation That Almost Wasn't

On December 29, 1972, I was just twelve years old and was supposed to be on a flight to Miami with my father and his second wife for a last minute winter getaway. It was an evening flight, leaving JFK International Airport in New York at 9:20. I was packed and ready to go, but a few days before the trip, I freaked out. I was having dreams about being wet, distinctly wet, in the cold, pitch black. I told Mom I would not get on that plane.

Dad was annoyed. (Okay, irate, but we'll go with annoyed for the sake of family harmony.) He told me I was being irrational, ridiculous and costing him a lot of money to change the reservations and miss another day of work. All true. I was sorry, but I would not get on that flight. As much as I loved my Dad, and really wanted to go to Florida, and would never, ever, intentionally cause him unhappiness, I would not budge. He could go without me. Dad called the next day and said he re-booked us on a flight the day before.

The next morning we woke up in our Miami condo to the devastating news that our original flight, Eastern Flight 401, had crashed in the everglades. It was the worst airline crash in South Florida's history. A chill went through the room. Dad looked at us and said, "I think that was our flight."

There is nothing rational about premonitions. Certain people will tell you they don't exist.

It's nice to think that everything in life is logical, yet the truth is, we live with a certain amount of uncertainty and magic.

Interestingly, there were fifty empty seats on that fateful flight to Miami, so perhaps I was not alone in sensing something and backing out at the last minute. Anyway, we did what any family would do having a close encounter with something terrifyingly unexplainable: we immediately put it out of our minds.

"Who wants to go swimming?" Dad asked.

Let Go and Let God

You cannot think yourself through close encounters of the unexplainable kind. There is no understanding why some survive an earthquake or a plane crash while others die. There is no explaining how certain people seem to possess a supernatural sensitivity, and others hear or see nothing unusual. For example, I can feel a certain type of energy in spaces or in people, while others think I might just be plain crazy. It just happens.

In yoga, B.K.S. Iyengar told us we should rely on love and devotion. I instead tend to think a lot. Most days on the mat, *my mind does not shut up.* I have to train my mind like a laser beam on a certain point of the practice, such as alignment or breath, if I have any hope to get any peace and quiet by the time it's naptime or *Savasana.*

There are many kinds of yoga for every kind of seeker from the highly analytical to the purely playful. Mr. Iyengar's style of practice was exacting, where instructors often spend an hour teaching one pose through props and cues. On the other end, there are Vinyasa styles where the instructor might ask you to get in touch with your inner ballerina or warrior goddess.

I am a fan of yoga aligned with a theme where the discipline of a very exacting practice is combined with a dose of inspiration or yoga perspective. As a teacher, I strive to find the balance of devotion with an analytical approach. I learned a series of physical directives that when systematically performed, enabled the student to be safe and go deeper into their practice: soften, hug, widen, tuck and extend. There are also energy loops and spirals. Soften, hug, widen, tuck and extend, then move this back, that forward, and puff, melt, puff again if necessary, same with melt, then scoop, firm and offer out. Over and over. For an obsessive-compulsive yogi like me, it is a dream come true. I am a happy little pig in you know what when I'm on my mat in an alignment class. Not even a sale at Nordstrom's could drag me out.

At the opposite end of the spectrum, Power Yoga relies more on feeling your way through the yoga with a flow of linked postures. Moving from one posture to the next with the momentum of breath prevents the mind from obsessing. You have to move it or you will lose it.

"Think less, be more."

Baron Baptiste said that. He brought Power Yoga to its current popularity in the United States. He explains in his book, *Journey into Power* that you have to get your brain out of the way to give your body and soul a chance to shine. Baptiste coined the phrase, "analysis paralysis," and he is truly speaking to me with that one. I have to be careful with the analysis I generate, so I do not create a paralysis in my practice.

"Let go and let God," quipped Ross Rayburn during a teacher training in New York in 2010. There is a point, Rayburn said, where all the preparation and practice, where the theory and principles will not carry you. And you'll have to trust that the Universe is going to carry you through. Easier said than done.

The Year I Lost My *Pincha*

Even if you know the way along a well-marked path, you can get lost.

I had a year in which I was lost on just the seventy-two inches of my mat. After eight years of practicing yoga on a daily basis, I suddenly could no longer do several arm balances and inversions. One day, I fell disastrously in Crow, *Bakasana* and almost broke my nose. The studio had a tightly woven carpet and after I fell, I slipped forward off my mat and got a nasty red rug burn down the center of my face.

"Why, hello there, Pepe Le Pew," my husband Mike said when I returned home, more than slightly mortified. "Maybe it's time we give this up and make dinner for a change?"

Even though I had fallen, I was not at all afraid to try it again. I was more cautious, but not more afraid. So when I lost one of my favorite poses, Forearm Stand, *Pincha Mayurasana*, there was no explaining it. In fact, if I had a signature pose, something I could count on, it would be *Pincha*. And it left me suddenly, like a good-looking stranger on a Sunday morning. *Wham bam*, gone.

Losing the pose began with an Immersion class. After practicing various kinds of yoga for seven years, I thought I'd try something new. This Immersion was 108 long hours and when you emerge, you realize you have been changed. Your practice is better and your heart is stronger. After so many years of stumbling through yoga, I was no longer an accidental yogi. I was filled with intention and I had finally learned how to do the poses correctly. But I also became mildly obsessive-compulsive with alignment. I immersed not just my practice, but my entire mind, heart and soul into the *how* of yoga.

Every time I came to a pose, I was practicing soften, hug, widen, tuck, extend, move back, forward, puff, melt, scoop, firm and drag. Over and over. I looked like a convulsive robot.

"Um, excuse me," my local teacher asked when I came back to practice, "but what on Earth are you doing?"

"I'm finding my alignment," I moaned.

"Really? Why don't you try being at ease?"

I'm thinking, *Why don't* you *try being middle-aged with arthritis, a hangover, massive fear, severe tightness, a pain in the butt and a bit of a wobbly belly and see how that's working for you.* But I said, "Thank you" instead.

Until that year, I had so much pride around the arm balances. While I struggled with anything that required flexibility, I could rock the strength postures. I could do certain moves that no respectable little old lady living in the Midwest should be able to do. Several of these moves are good for yoga party tricks, although I learned the hard way that friends don't let friends drink and invert.

I loved these poses because of the sense of freedom and strength I had. Yet for years I never analyzed it. I just did it. And more often than not, it worked. When I re-learned how to do the postures with the proper alignment, I began to understand the mechanics and the meaning in my body. It was thrilling, but certain things were going to have to change.

The first posture I had to change completely was Headstand, *Sirsasana*. It turned out I had been doing it wrong. Who knew? My teacher Amy Ippoliti knew, and apparently my body did as well, which is why I got a resounding headache every time I practiced it. I just never listened to my body before. Amy is harder to ignore.

"No, no, no," she said, as she repositioned my head further forward, nearer the hairline on the floor. I could just see her toes in my upside down peripheral vision as she stood by watching me and everyone else tottering on our heads. Even if she wasn't standing next to you, she had her eye on you. From across a crowded room, she could see if the bottom of my wrists were lacking engagement on the floor. "Meeeechelle" she would project across the room, "Wrists." She has the eyes of a hawk, I swear.

Now that I was doing the pose correctly and without pain, for some reason I suddenly could not do it at all. Nowadays, I realize it's common that when a student changes his alignment it may take time to adjust. Just because something seems counterintuitive, does not mean it is wrong. It could be a change for the better and we are just not yet used to it. Nevertheless, I was struggling. Everything looked good, but for some reason, I could no longer balance. My habit of the old alignment was so ingrained that I could not find steadiness in the new version.

A few weeks after the Immersion, I still could not do Headstand. However, I was scheduled to teach an inversion workshop with my yoga friend and fellow teacher, Michelle, the younger, thinner, taller, blonder Michelle of *Colorado*. When we agreed to do the workshop, I was a "master of inversions" (ironically, when I didn't actually know what I was doing). Now, I could no longer do Headstand and felt like a student again, but I needed to take the teacher's seat very soon for this workshop. When I told Michelle I could no longer do Headstand, she said, "Well, you've got exactly three weeks to fix that."

And so I did. In two weeks and five days, I found my new Headstand. I came, I saw, I conquered. I got up, I stayed up, and we taught the workshop brilliantly.

That is why when I lost Forearm Stand, *Pincha Mayurasana*, and I could neither come up nor balance, I was thinking I could fix it in two weeks and maybe four days. I have always been very strong in this pose. In the Immersion, we did a timed forearm stand against a wall; when I was in the correct alignment, I beat nearly the whole room hanging in there for almost six minutes. That's one for the old people!

But all of a sudden, I couldn't do it at all.

For some reason, I was terrified. Fear swept over me like a volcanic rush of mud and ash and pinned me down to the mat. I could not rise up from the muck.

I lost this posture at the end of January 2008. Two weeks went by. Nothing. I focused on Michelle's words like a mantra, "You've got three weeks to fix that." Nothing. I sought out a million different teachers who each tried different techniques. I meditated. I visualized. I wrote in my yoga journal. Nothing. I tried acupuncture and considered hypnotism. Nothing.

I had completely lost it.

February.

March.

April.

May.

This lasted eighteen months!

I worked with a brick. I worked at the wall. I prayed to God, and then to Ganesha, the Elephant deity who removes obstacles. I even offered God a trade that if he brought back my *Pincha Mayurasana*, I would no longer curse, especially with my kids. Nothing. Okay, maybe I'll give up drinking? Nothing. Or give up chips and dip? Nothing. I wore a crystal necklace for courage, and one for healing, and one for stability. My neck was almost sore from all the crystals, but still no pose. Nada. Goose eggs.

Then one day I was in a yoga class at the back of the room. The teacher asked for Dolphin Pose, which could be the set up to *Pincha*.

And instead of practicing soften, hug, widen, tuck, extend, move back, forward, puff, melt, scoop, firm and drag, this is what I did: I said, *"Fuck it."*

"I give up," I told God.

And up I went. I came, I rose, I conquered. I could not believe it and started to cry. Let me tell you, I will never take that posture, *or any posture*, for granted again.

Ross Rayburn is right. At a certain point, all the training and education has to make room for that 99% of practice, love and devotion. Praise the Lord!

A Lesson From the Mat

Grace Is the Answer

Grace is not just the bigger picture. Grace *is* the picture.

If analysis paralysis is getting too much into the details, then Grace is the 99% whirling around us that we cannot think our way through. You cannot think your way through to Grace. You have to feel it.

Sometimes I see a student and I'm trying to figure out why he or she cannot do a certain pose. I'm looking and looking at the body and the alignment. Though I try, I cannot see what is holding them back. It is the same thing with teaching a class. Sometimes I enter a room and I can't put my finger on it, but something is off. The energy, the breath, the feeling, it is off. Staring at each student often does not provide the answer. Instead, I have to pull back and take a bigger view.

When the answers are not apparent in the details, you need to step back. I have seen teachers trying to get in touch with something bigger. You need to consider not just the student, but also some bigger energy. I have seen teachers hold a person in an inversion, and close their eyes to *feel the way* to the person's alignment.

In order to see the bigger picture, you might have to shield your vision from the obvious. To gain clarity, you need to see the whole picture. Try to take a big view, of yourself, of the alignment and the energy, and then get in touch with the magic around it. That's Grace.

A Lesson From the Mat

When the How Becomes the Now

How do we know when we are ready? How do we know when we have the skill, but we need confidence? Or faith? Yoga is not like a university, when one day someone hands you a diploma and says, "You are now ready to go upside down in the middle of the room." It is a subtle, moving target, this thing called readiness.

"The answer to how, is always now," said Baron Baptiste.

He was in Denver teaching a roomful of anxious type "A" yogis, and the theme today was about taking the plunge and moving ahead with your life. "If you are really ready," he said, "you don't need the 'how.' If you are not ready, the how becomes the now."

But I like the "how," I'm thinking. The "how" is pretty good. And without the "how," how will I know if I am ready? (I am sort of whining here.)

"Don't worry about the technique," I heard in a conference in Colorado. "It will come. The attitude is more important."

But when? I'm waiting! (More whining.) *Somebody tell me when.*

"Everything that holds us back has the potential to set us free," explained my teacher in one of his local classes in Denver.

Okay. You people are seriously bugging me here.

A Lesson From the Mat

Working Through a Plateau

This is very unconventional advice. But if you hit a plateau in your practice, if you have tried everything, sought out advice, paid for privates and nothing is working, try this: Forget about it and move on. Chances are you will be completely happy and content in the world without the pose.

And chances are that is when you will get it.

I know this makes no sense. But there are lots of things in life that make no sense. The sooner you get comfortable with how little life makes sense, the sooner you will find yourself gliding through the rough spots.

As soon as I tossed out the possibility of getting Handstand, I became free from a paralyzing part of my practice. I would tell myself, I have a great husband, healthy and wonderful kids, a nice cozy home, crazy but good dogs. I can live happily without this pose. And guess what?

I know, right? It makes no sense. That's what I'm trying to tell you.

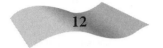

Quiet the Mind

Yoga is the cessation of the fluctuations of the mind.
Then the seer dwells in his own true splendor.
~ The Yoga Sutras of Patanjali

You must shut up to listen. That explains why yoga is hard for me: I am very good at talking.

If you can't get quiet, you can't clear away the clutter in your mind. If you can't find space, there is no room for anything new. Therefore, to listen, to grow wiser, you must eventually *shut the fuck up.* That is my loose interpretation of the Yoga Sutras 1.2 and 1.3.

It often takes a great shout from the Universe to get my attention, to get me to take note. I can ignore pain, or rush around like a crazy woman ignoring my health, until something happens that I cannot disregard. Like trying to do a Downward Facing Dog, *Adho Mukha Svanasana* with a separated shoulder. That was bad. Or having a heart attack. A heart attack will get my attention.

One night while driving carpool I believed I was having a heart attack. I am totally serious. I had a pain in my chest so severe I had to pull over the car.

This was when my boys were 14 and 15, and each had a million activities that often kept us on the road as late as 10:00

after a sports event. I would wake up at 5:30 in the morning because I had to drive my son to high school at 6:30, unless he had basketball practice, which meant he had to be at school by 5:30 A.M. *I cannot make this stuff up.* When most people are sleeping, our early mornings were a blur of breakfast, packing lunches, planning pick up and afternoon activities, last minute homework, feeding the dogs, and so on. I know there is a reader out there who is saying, *she should pack those lunches at night and get better organized,* and to that I say, with all the love in my heart, thank you! (You know what I really wanted to say, but I am further along to enlightenment now, so I say "thank you" instead.)

During the day I would prepare my classes, teach, practice, do laundry, shop for groceries, volunteer for school as

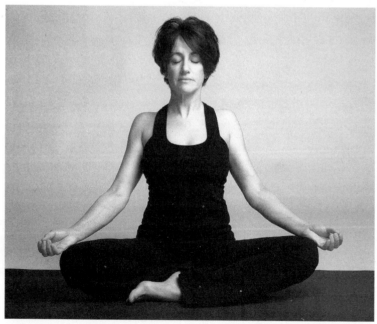

Pose: Meditation Seat, *Sukhasana.* Trying to look good at this!

minimally as I could get away with, attempt to make dinner, or at least buy it somewhere, and care for aging parents. Everything it takes to keep a household running. Then, I would pick up the kids and go to soccer, basketball, music, the orthodontist. (You see the orthodontist so much in these years you could practically be having an affair!) If I had a microwave in my minivan, I'd never have to leave the van.

"The funny part about being really busy," said a friend of mine, "is that people who don't know what it is to be busy think they are busier than the rest of us." This friend is the director of a national arts foundation, works full time, and manages her home, including two stepchildren, with little to no help. (Sorry, but her husband, whom I adore, just doesn't count as help.) Then, for her fiftieth birthday, she decided to go back to school full time and earn a master's degree. An Ivy League master's degree. No slacking allowed.

"Everyone thinks they are the busiest," she commented. "And pointing out that they don't work, or don't have children, or only have one day a week where they don't have the maid, just doesn't help."

Busy is a state of mind.

Or is it that you are only as busy as you think you are?

But trying to keep up with an insane schedule can also get your attention. Here I am, driving on the freeway, trying to get my son to soccer practice. And we are late, of course. We are late because after a day of work I picked him up from school—late. I fed him, changed clothes, packed soccer gear, and picked up my younger son—late. I threw them both in the car with snack and homework, locked up the dogs, ran out, and now we are all worried that the older one will be late to practice, which could mean less playing time. The traffic is not moving. And I am having a heart attack.

My chest gets so tight it feels like a stabbing pain. I cannot breathe. I try to use my yoga breath, counting to four, then six, but it's not working. (Funny, it didn't work in childbirth either.) So I turn off the blaring rap music and tell the kids I don't feel well. Twenty minutes later we are still inching along the highway, so I explain to my boys what to do if I pass out. Remember that CPR training you had? And don't forget to call 911. And please God take my ashes back to the East Coast where I belong.

When nothing else works, a heart attack will get my attention. In my car, I am finally taking note. It turns out I did not have a heart attack, but whatever it was that night on the freeway, stress or heartburn, I finally listened. I cannot, and will not, do it all. But most importantly:

I suddenly understood: *I am not that busy!*

I was not so busy that it was worth dying on a Colorado highway! Even if I have a million things to do on the outside, I will no longer be busy on the inside. I can choose my state of mind. I am in control of how to react to my schedule. Better yet, I can choose my schedule! I started cancelling classes, rearranging my teaching, making time to practice yoga, and telling everyone a whole lot of "no."

Clear Away the Noise

While there is no "I" in team, there is definitely an "I" in mind. The mind is often not on your team. It is a terrible team player.

In yoga, it is often the mind and not the body that is ready to quit. For example, when the teacher says, "Handstand," the mind often says, "Time to go to the bathroom."

"If your mind piped up just now and said you cannot do this, simply thank it for sharing and move on," said my friend Michelle.

"Yoga is the cessation of the fluctuations of the mind," according to the *Yoga Sutras of Patanjali*. When we succeed in our practice, the mind becomes still.

Of the triumvirate mind, body and soul, the mind can be the most irritating. Right when you need support, it chimes in with the most disparaging opinions, like a mother-in-law that never really liked you in the first place. "Oh you held a Handstand?" the mind says. "But for how long? No matter what you accomplish, the mind is quick to say, "You suck!"

To find out who we are, to delve into our true nature, we may have to get our mind out of the way. It is at best a distraction. At worst, it is a frenemy—not quite a friend, not quite an enemy.

But how do we learn to be quiet? Meditation.

You Always Remember the First

I had begun a meditation practice before my yoga Immersion. I would sit for five minutes after a class, or in the car, and it felt good. It is like a mini time-out from life. Once, the kids were fighting in Target and I lay down on the floor in *Savasana* and said I would not budge from my "meditation" until they worked it out. (Took about one minute.) So I was digging meditation.

In fact, I was good at *looking good at meditation.* After class, I would sit and make the finger *mudra* where Pointer and Thumbman touch in a circle. But in reality my head hung forward, my shoulders were rounded, my low back was so weak it practically sagged on the ground and the pain of sitting got me out of the pose in about thirty seconds. Still, it was probably long enough for everyone else to notice I was a "cool yogi."

Then in my Immersion, my teacher announced we would be working up to a thirty-minute meditation by the end of part three. This was terrifying to me. A half-hour meditation has about as much in common with a five minute sit, as say the World Series has with the Babe Ruth Little Sluggers. Only the outer form of the posture is the same. I felt like a five year old being thrown into the show.

Furthermore, I had a lot of very good reasons to avoid meditation:

- My back was not very strong and so it might hurt.
- I had no spare time as a busy mom, so if I was going to do something it should be multi-tasking, like getting a workout on the stair climber while calling my

best friend and simultaneously planning how not to make dinner.

- My nose was very itchy.
- I didn't have the right cushion. Or pants, or top, or little jewel for my forehead.
- I was not allowed to talk. *OMG!*

So I had a great deal of apprehension. Every day the teacher announced that we were going to do this monster meditation at the end of the week, and every day I would sit near the door and plan my escape.

We focused on breathing techniques, used the *bandhas*, or the internal binding methods for strength and support, and practiced opening the hips and strengthening the back. Then we chanted to quiet the mind.

Instead of inspiring confidence, the closer we got to the meditation, the more panicky I felt. Though we spent many hours sitting on a cushion on the ground, my back did not feel like it was getting stronger. I fidgeted and fussed. I took Advil at night. I griped to my husband that I wanted to quit, then Mike would give me the Marchildon pep talk about how we're not quitters, blah, blah, blah. But I am only a Marchildon by marriage, so maybe I could be a quitter, right?

"Berman," he'd say to me. (That's my maiden name.) "You are now a Marchildon and you need to man up. We don't quit."

The day for meditation finally arrived and we prepared to sit by placing cushions and straps, blocks and rugs wherever we needed extra support. I was trussed up like a chicken, and felt … comfortable? I was sure it wouldn't last, but at the moment, I was … okay.

Then my teacher got my attention. She said, once the mind is settled, amazing things can happen. You may hear voices or you may feel lighter, like an out-of-body experience. You can have visions. And sometimes, if you have a problem, the answer may come to you.

Now she really had my attention. Because if anyone had problems, it was me! With two pre-teens and a menopausal woman in the house, rational, reliable wisdom was in short supply. I instantly had a new attitude about this meditation. *Wooo hooo!* I felt the openness of Grace. If this practice could actually bring clarity into my life, I was prepared to sit until kingdom come.

So I closed my eyes and let everything go, because this is what I know for sure: All that stuff, all that junk you have to do, the laundry, kids, carpool, *it will still be there after you meditate.* Even if you sit for thirty minutes, you won't be missing a thing! The sit lasted through several stages, and when the thirty minutes were up, it was the most beautiful feeling you can imagine.

In meditation, I felt more connected to the world.

It was an incredible feeling of belonging to the Universe, even to nature. And up to that moment, I'd felt that nature was something that needed to be swept out of the kitchen once a day when the dogs tracked it inside.

Furthermore, I had a vision, and I even heard voices (I hope my family is not reading this part of the book because they will surely commit me now). I had several immediate problems looming in my life, and now I seemed to have the solutions. If you sit and be quiet, if you can clear away all the clutter so you can focus the mind, if the mind then wanders until it seems to focus, then the answers have an opportunity to appear. It is like shining a flashlight in the dark; we get a glimpse of light that can lead the way.

After this meditation, I called Mike. I told him that I had I found peace and calm. And better yet, I knew how to handle several of the issues that had weighed down our family. He was thrilled that my newfound wisdom did not involve a trip to the mall, which is how I used to solve most of my problems.

Withdraw to Connect

From Hamlet to Shiva, every religion, culture and mythology includes a time when one withdraws from the world to find themselves. Wandering in the woods, sitting in a cave, sailing at sea are all forms of withdrawing from daily life. The Quakers say, "We sit together in silence to listen for that still small voice within." Even Jesus instructed, "Be still and know that I Am."

All the craziness running from here to there does not contribute one iota to wisdom. In fact, it detracts. I am convinced it is how we run away from the things we don't want to know. I'd like to write on my son's college application that when he gave up the clarinet in high school, he had more time to sit silently everyday to reflect on absolutely nothing at all, and he seemed much happier and more grounded than before. Ha!

It's hard to explain, but practicing a disengaged consciousness actually helps to focus the consciousness. Or practicing non-attachment in meditation actually increases the feeling of connectedness to community. The ego's imagined barriers between self and others seem to melt away. As Patanjali said, when the mind becomes quiet, the seer dwells in his true splendor. The noise clears away, and what is left is self-knowledge, the ultimate goal of yoga.

Another way to put it is, when you meditate, you see life from a bigger perspective. The "to do" list fades away and it's more about the "to be" list. It is about moving your practice more toward the bigger picture of love and devotion, rather than seeing from the channel of *"whatsinitforme."*

Meditation allows you to "know yourself as a spirit and not just a thing," writes Deepak Chopra in his book, *Ageless Body, Timeless Mind*. Chopra documents that there is a physical reaction to meditation; it has been shown to lower levels of cortisol and adrenaline and reduce stress. In fact, he says that regular meditators show a substantial reduction in three markers for human aging: blood pressure, near point vision loss and hearing loss.

So next time you are really, really busy, perhaps even having a potential heart attack on the way to soccer practice, try doing less, not more. Ask yourself, how busy are you really? Try sitting still for just five minutes.

The highest purpose of gaining wisdom in our lives is to align ourselves with the Universe. When we are aligned, life feels effortless. When we are misaligned, we struggle. "When you pray, you *ask* the Universe," explains my friend and yoga teacher Heather Peterson. "When you meditate, you *listen*. It's all the same conversation." Maybe it's time to listen for a change?

A Lesson From the Mat

Why Ganesha Rides the Mouse

Why does Hinduism's largest God ride the world's smallest animal?

There are different interpretations for why Lord Ganesha, a giant, portly figure with an elephant head, rides a teeny, tiny mouse. Every deity has a ride; it could be a white bull, or a swan, or a peacock. But Ganesha balances his huge frame on top of a mouse. Some myths say it is because elephants are afraid of mice, so Ganesha keeps a reminder of his fear nearby. Other myths explain that it is because the mouse is a symbol of the mind. The mind is like a mouse, making an incessant chattering as it nibbles and busies its way through life. So does the mind; it is rarely quiet and peaceful.

Perhaps it is for both reasons. Ganesha rides the mouse as a symbol of overcoming his fear, and to support his steady effort to override the mind's chatter. Just as we need to remind ourselves continuously we are more than our thoughts or fears, Ganesha too, is a symbol of how even the most powerful Gods fight the same battle as we mortals driving carpool. See, we are not alone!

A Lesson From the Mat

The Thinking Bath

I hear voices, and sometimes they are loud.

Never having been predisposed to schizophrenia, I was surprised to find that during menopause I was suddenly besieged by voices in my head. They would come out of nowhere, having full-blown conversations that I could not stop. They would wake me up at night, distract me while driving, and worst of all, interrupt my yoga practice.

I was alarmed. Who are these people and why are they taking up so much space in my head?

"When you are overwhelmed by thoughts," explained my teacher, "Sometimes you need to take a thinking bath."

Rather than running away from the things on your mind, the answer may be to go deeper in. Next time you are overwhelmed by your thoughts, stop what you are doing, and concentrate instead. If the voices woke you up, write everything down in a journal, then try to go back to sleep. If the voices show up while you are driving or running errands, carry a pad of paper and write the thoughts down. If you are meditating, breathe and focus on each thought through to the end. By taking a deep, long soak in your thoughts, you might be able to release them like popping bubbles in a bath.

A Lesson From the Mat

Meditation ABC's

Meditating is hard, but it doesn't have to be. There are certain techniques to make it more accessible to those of us who spend our days driving cars or sitting at desks.

- Warm up with a deep stretch to open your hips, back and shoulders.
- Make sure your position is comfortable. The knees need to be level or below the hips with the feet folded in front. You may need a cushion or a blanket to elevate your seat.
- If your low back needs more support, you can lean against a wall or sit in a chair.
- Keep your posture tall. Good posture is easier to maintain than bad. Bring the chin slightly back so the head does not hang forward. Keep the heart lifted as a sign of your intention to stay bright.
- Start small. Go for five minutes at first and then gradually increase your time.
- At first, breathe consciously. See if you can stretch the breath to six counts. Later in the meditation you can let the breath become a natural rhythm.
- Find a mantra to focus the mind. *"Om Namah Shivaya"* works. "Please God give me the strength to see the good in my teenagers, love my mother-in-law,

and not kill my husband," is too long to fit within a single breath.

- As you ease into the meditation, you will be able to let go of the counting, the mantra and the jumble of thoughts in your mind so you can feel a single point of consciousness, a oneness with the Universe, like a guiding light. Congratulations.

PART THREE

Growing Stronger

Taking Action in Our Lives

Dream big, for a dream leads us to reality. If you have no dreams, no desire or even a foolish aspiration for something more in your life, then you have no guiding light.

The third part of the journey is taking action in life. Action is the realization of our dreams. It is when we take our fearless heart, lifted by the wisdom we've gained, to live stronger on and off the mat.

Growing stronger is about who you are, and who you were meant to be. It's realizing you don't have anything to prove, especially to the younger, thinner person on the mat next to you, unless you want to prove something to yourself. It's about discovering how to make a difference in the world so you leave a legacy for the ones you love. It's about standing up for the things you believe in, and showing others by example. It's about finding your dharma, your true calling, and living it. It's about finding your inner badass.

Yoga is the invitation to live up to our potential. The mat becomes a catalyst for transformation. Practicing becomes our path, where we grow not just older, but better, wiser and stronger. We become so much more in our lives, for ourselves, and for those we love, every time we offer ourselves to something greater. This is the promise of yoga: it is the promise of more.

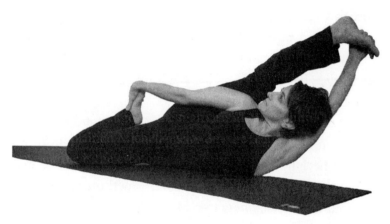

Lizard Pose, *Utthan Pristhasana,* variation. Who's a badass now?

13

Find Your Inner Badass

Our deepest fear is not that we are inadequate.
Our deepest fear is that we are powerful beyond measure.
~ Marianne Williamson

"Sometimes you need to be a bitch to get things done," Madonna said.

My secret is this: I can be a bitch.

I wasn't always this way. I spent some time playing nice. Even when I worked in a cutthroat marketing job at a Fortune 100 company, I played nice. I smiled when the guy from the next cubicle over took my job because by then I was a working mom and everyone knew that working mothers don't have the energy or time to fight back. I allowed others to take credit for my work because they probably needed it more than I did. When issues came up, I'd say, "That's okay." I mean, I am the girl who lay down in a bathroom and decided not to fight but to survive and clean up the mess instead. I can be very accommodating.

Although I was good at playing nice, it just wasn't me. I was meant to be large and in charge. The confusing thing is that I come in a small package. This puzzled even me for a while. I thought I needed to be sweet or a little weak to be a girl.

It was certainly confusing to my ex-husband. In my first marriage, I was deeply lost in the land of "nice."

Right after our honeymoon we moved to Cincinnati where as a couple of writers, we had plenty of imagination but never enough money. We needed a better car, one that would actually start in the morning. We needed a place to live. We needed to eat, for Christ's sake! So I did what anyone would do; I left journalism, went corporate and made us some money. And while I was commuting an hour a day to work, he was busy checking out of the marriage.

I was not blameless in this thing, as is usually the case, because most of all, I'm not sure if he was ever really married to me. Instead, he was married to my Nice Girl Avatar, who was super sweet, trying to cook and clean, work full time, and praise him constantly. Not once if he said he was hungry, did I tell him to get off his ass and make himself something to eat. Not once! Or pick up his clothes. Or do his own laundry. *What the hell?*

A part of me was always afraid that this marriage between the Writer and the Nice Girl was going to blow up. I was trying so hard to be someone else that it was like living as a spy. What if he found out? And then after he announced that he was leaving me and moving to the other side of the country because he found his true love, and that he was taking everything; and by the way, he had never loved me, and I had absolutely nothing but my ten-year-old cocker spaniel and a food processor I did not know how to use, after all that, he said he had known the truth about me all along.

We were sitting in a family counselor's office, which is what you do when you are from New York and your spouse announces he is leaving you: you seek counseling. And the therapist asked my ex if he was worried about leaving me with pretty much nothing.

"I'm not worried about Michelle," he said. "She is very competent. (Pause.)

V-e-r-y Com-pe-tent. She will be fine."

He had me, as he'd liked to say, *dead to rights.*

So you see, he knew. My dirty little secret was now out in the open: I am competent. If fact, I might be one of the most capable people in the world, and it cost me my marriage.

My mother and grandmother were two of the most accomplished and intelligent women and I was right there with them. I was raised to do as they had done, stand on my own two feet. Growing up, one of the most valued possessions we owned was a toolbox my mother had been refining for years. I might be a girl, but I knew how to fix most things around a house or boat. No matter how much my mother loved and depended on the toolbox, when she met the ex-husband, she took one look at him and decided I might be up a creek, so to speak.

"You're going to need it more than me," she said, handing over the sacred metal box on my wedding day. Her gift to me was self-sufficiency.

If I was competent, if I was strong and capable, rather than hiding these gifts, maybe it was time to step up and ring the bell? Maybe it was time to own my power? Although I didn't know it at the time, I would survive this divorce. I'd go on to date men ten years younger to ten years older: lawyers, writers, architects and more. I travelled, I found a new career, and then another. And then one day, I met a man who instead of trying to hold me back, said, "You go baby. Show 'em what you can do." So I married him.

I was strong, powerful, competent, intelligent, and good-looking, too. And what my ex intended when he said I was competent was he meant I was a bitch. It was my truth and my deepest fear.

Who Are We, Really?

Years later, I was on my yoga mat and the bitch was pretty much gone. Yet, I am a mom, and anyone who's ever been a parent knows that the last thing you feel is competent. You doubt yourself at every turn. I had already started a therapy fund for my kids.

I am sorry to admit, I have at times not been the best parent. I have spanked them (not terribly hard), yelled at them (occasionally), thrown dishes, cried at length, and placed myself in time-outs. (It was useless for the kids, but very effective for me, with a glass of wine, and the Oprah show.) From me, they learned the "F" word when they were two, and that ketchup is a vegetable. (Ronald Reagan was right, and on a McDonald's hamburger it definitely created a well-balanced meal.) I allowed them to eat the school lunches and ride the school bus since kindergarten.

And I never joined them for lunch in the cafeteria or played with them at recess in school like many of the mothers in my neighborhood. (OMG! Can you even imagine?) I have never done their homework. I have rarely fought their battles. But on occasion, if they were grossly outnumbered or outplayed by an adult—and there are lots of adults that take advantage of kids I'm sorry to say—I have stepped in.

And when I did, it was usually ugly. Therefore, my kids are becoming adept at fighting their own battles in a much more diplomatic way.

In general, I have allowed my sons to live their own lives, and make their own mistakes, which is not the norm these days. However, my boys also know I love them to death and I will do absolutely anything for them.

Unconditional love is priceless.

Better yet, I have unconditional faith in their abilities to do anything they want. I believe wholly in their potential and I'm here to support it.

Yet by the time I arrived on my yoga mat in my forties, the competent go-getter woman of my youth was really just very tired. Exhausted in fact. I was overweight, out of shape, and I had lost my edge. I was on the work-family merry-go-round and I was slightly nauseous. It was in this condition that my teacher asked me to find "my inner badass."

"My what?"

"Your inner badass," she said. "Show me your light."

And just like that, I decided that if my inner badass had gone to sleep, it might be time to wake it up. I went looking for the strong, competent woman I used to be, and I found her in the strengthening arm balances of yoga. More than anything else, these poses saved me. I didn't have the flexibility to touch my toes, but I could do *Bakasana*, Crow. My spine was so rounded that I could not move my shoulder blades onto my back, but I could do *Eka Pada Koundinyasana II*, the Hurdles.

As I started to build my strength on the mat, a light also went on inside me. I began to walk a little taller and step a little brighter into the world. I returned to the mat not just to find a stronger butt, but a stronger life. I looked to regain the person I was meant to be: a strong, powerful, competent, enormously intelligent and beautiful woman. And if that is what society calls a bitch, then so be it. *My haters can suck it!*

When you decide it is time to live your best life, it will be time to embrace every aspect of your quirky personality, the good and the bad.

**Living stronger
requires a radical acceptance of the self.**

And then, with perspective, you might see that the parts of yourself you considered your weaknesses, are actually also your strengths. My competency may have cost me a marriage, but it is now the thing that makes me great. You cannot hide forever. And when you come out of your own closet, you will be brilliant. You will live a little louder. This is living stronger.

A Lesson From the Mat

Don't Wait for Fifty

There is something wild and crazy that happens when many of us turn fifty. We don't give a hoot about what people think anymore. We are set free in a way that is exhilarating.

Suzanne Braun Levine in her book, *Fifty Is the New Fifty*, coined this new attitude of knowing who you are and what you want, and not caring what others think, "*The Fuck You Fifties.*" We reach a point where we know ourselves and we finally become awake to our potential. We have earned a sense of mastery. We know we can handle what life throws at us. We've taken risks, we've found some rewards, and we're moving on to new adventures.

In my case, my children are growing and starting to drive to their own activities, and I am getting used to spending time with me, on my mat. With any luck, when this happens we will like what we see. Holding back from living fully is no longer polite. It isn't authentic. It's just our fear of being great.

My hope is that we don't have to wait until we're fifty to discover who we are. The opportunity is always there. When we make some small accomplishment on our yoga mat, it's a chance to take another step forward in our life. You can start whenever you're ready; you don't have to wait for permission, or for a certain age. You can go for it now.

A Lesson From the Mat

The Honey Badger Is a Badass

In fact, this little badger is known as being among the baddest badasses in the world. It knows what it wants, and it goes after it. It loves honey, and so it can withstand a thousand bee stings to get it. It can tolerate the venom of the cobra to be one of the snake's few natural predators. As the Internet star Randall (who narrates a video about the honey badger) says, this animal doesn't give a shit! It is one tough mother.

It's good to be a bit of a honey badger and go after what we want in our lives and let nothing get in our way. We develop perseverance. Yet, the honey badger is so badass, it might be a little lonely. This mammal finds it difficult to mate, it suffers from a naturally low birth rate, and when it does have babies, it often eats its young. If we ultimately want successful relationships, we may have to curb our inner honey badger to get along, and I certainly don't recommend eating our young, unless they are teenagers.

A Lesson From the Mat

Arm Balances Are Badass

I love balancing on my arms. It is in the arm balances where I can let my inner badass shine.

While many of the arm balances are about art and architecture—knowing what goes where—there is also a certain amount of strength and courage involved. Nothing feels better than knocking out an arm balance. And nothing feels worse or more self-defeating, than the days when I am too tired to haul my *"ass-ana"* up there.

The secret is being content with whatever it is you can bring to your mat. Some days are better than others. That, to me, is the real power of arm balances. They simply let us know where we are at the moment and teach us to have both strength and compassion in our practice.

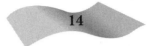

14

Breaking the
Spell of Mortality

I don't want the normal human experience.
~ Desiree Rumbaugh

On the day the "Rapture" was predicted (which was supposed to be the end of the world), I am on a plane. Of course, I am. That's my luck! Thank God there's a bar cart coming around.

I hate to whine, but I am not a good flyer. I try, but I'm not always brave. It's part of the human experience to be a gutless, spineless wreck sometimes, and right now I keep imagining that the world below me, including everyone I love, will vaporize before my eyes. I wish I was more like James Bond; whenever he was facing certain death he was still able to enjoy a martini, shaken not stirred. Nothing rattled him.

As strong as we are, we can still find ourselves clinging to the things we are afraid to lose, you know, like our lives. I've been practicing yoga for more than a decade and at the end of the day, the lesson of non-clinging is hard. As humans, we tend to hang on tight to what we've got. Unfortunately, clinging to what you have means you make no room for anything new. Nevertheless, right now, I'm very interested in staying alive. So I'll take a pomegranate martini from the bar cart while I'm waiting to see how this Rapture thing turns out.

Make Room For More

One lesson of yoga is that you must clean out the old in order to fill up with something new. The jeans in the store might be fabulous, but you need to make room in your closet to hang them. On a more spiritual note, you need to clear away old, self-defeating thoughts to fill up with new empowering thoughts. You need to clear away bad habits and misalignments before you can make changes in your practice. And you need to clear out all the little disappointments and hurts in your heart to have room for a new and stronger love. Seriously.

**You have to get rid of the things
that are no longer serving you.**

It's like bad bathing suits you never should have bought. Get rid of that shit. It's the same in life.

A lifetime ago, I made a promise to myself that I was going to get up, brush myself off, and live extremely well. Ridiculously well. I was going to fall in love, have a family, do something rewarding and wear designer jeans. I was not going to let the past have one iota of influence on how my future was going to be. I knew there were good men out there; I just had to find them. So once I was old enough to be legally transported across state lines, I began an all out pursuit of good looking, wonderful, kind, and talented men. Especially good looking. Did I mention that?

Given my rough start, I was surprisingly adept at dating. I have dated all kinds of men: journalists, cowboys, architects, artists, lawyers, and businessmen. I have dated long-haired, short-haired, and no-haired men. I have dated thin men, short men, tall men, and strong men. And I can say this with absolute certainty: *I loved most every one of them.*

I am not sure why I always had a full dance card. But it could be because of two things. Number one: I made a point of love. Number two: I never held on to any of them too tightly.

Being able to love is a skill, I believe, that not many people today possess. These days people are able to hook up, hang out, and chill but they are not able or willing to love. They struggle to say the words. They are reluctant to commit. By floating along the surface and never diving down deep, they actually experience less of the ocean of emotion. They limit themselves.

I am going to guess that most of us learned how to love from those who loved us, and thankfully, I learned from my Mom. Mom is the most loving and giving person on earth. She taught me my first lesson on love:

Love is abundant; there is never any end to it.

The more I screwed up, the more she loved me. The more I frustrated or aggravated her, the more she loved me. The more I loved her back, the more she loved me. It was never ending. In fact, she is so loving she can be downright embarrassing at times, hugging and kissing me for way too long especially in public, but still, there was never any question that I was loved.

The second reason I had a full dance card was I valued my freedom. I believed that saying about fish in the sea. I could love completely, but I could also let it go just as easily. It seems that these days the more typical human experience includes cyber-stalking our exes. Friends, listen up: non-clinging drives the opposite sex wild.

Hold On Lightly

Of course this works both ways. So the one who held on the least to me is the one who taught me the lesson of non-clinging.

We met when I was just five years old, and he was, maybe ten. I was hanging upside down from a tree with my flowered underpants showing, and he said he knew then, he wanted to marry me. Right? This is very romantic.

Mr. Knightley, we'll call him, lived down the street from my favorite cousins—three rambunctious boys who would spend the weekends torturing me. They would lure me outside where I'd be the monkey in the middle, they'd help me climb a tree only to run away and leave me screaming for help, or they'd persuade me to go inside and get some treats from my aunt, then steal them out of my hands. The worst was when they'd talk me into "Red Light, Green Light," and after I had counted to ten, I'd turn around to see absolutely nothing—no boys, no friends; even the dog had left me. I'd be standing there bawling my eyes out and then Mr. Knightley would appear in my backyard. He'd get me down from the tree or help me find my cousins. One day, he looked into my eyes and said, "I'm going to marry you."

Of course it didn't work out like that. High school then college sent us both in different directions and I did not see him for twenty years. Then came the day of my cousin's wedding and by then, he was a lawyer and I was a journalist. He asked me to dance and it was ridiculous. RIDICULOUS. I fell so hard for him that for the first time in my life, I could not eat. I could not sleep. *I could barely breathe.* I did not know what had come over me, because truthfully, I had not lost sleep over any man in my entire life.

We started to date, yet we lived in two different states and had two very different lives. I was a greenhorn journalist bouncing from paper to paper, from town to town. He was establishing his practice in New Orleans. He said he would never ask me to leave my career for him. Right? Why would I want to leave a low-paying job working fourteen-hour days and living with cockroaches, when I could be with the one I loved who happened to be a successful lawyer? *What on earth is wrong with us when we're young?* He wanted me; I wanted my career. We drifted apart.

Five years later my career had taken me to writing for the morning newspaper in Birmingham, Alabama, just a few hours from New Orleans. But although I wasn't dating anyone seriously, I was afraid to call Mr. Knightley. I thought, he's probably married by now. He may not even remember my name.

And then, the Universe stepped in. A friend won a trip to New Orleans for the weekend and he invited me to come along. After a night on the town, we stopped into an all-night diner for a bite to eat at 2:00 A.M. The server seated us at the counter, and when I looked to my left, Mr. Knightley was sitting right next to me! *I cannot make this stuff up.* My arm brushed his. I looked at Knightley, and he at me, and I said,

"I'm really not with 'him,'" thumbing to my date. I went home with Mr. Knightley and we began phase two of our romance.

This time I thought for sure we would get married. After a year I was hoping for a ring, but I got a relocation proposal instead. He asked me to consider moving to New Orleans, but I did not have a job there that worked for me. So again, we drifted apart. I married someone else, and so did he. I divorced, and so did he. I changed careers and now worked as a speechwriter in an office cubicle in Dayton, Ohio. About a year after my divorce, with no one in my life except my elderly cocker spaniel, I thought of Mr. Knightley. I was done with the old patterns, the old loves, and the old stupid shit that we do to ourselves. I was ready for new. Would he like to meet for a drink?

Then it was on. After three false starts, we were ready. We met everywhere we could: Dayton, Memphis, New York, New Orleans. Things were humming along. I wasn't ultra clingy, but I wasn't ultra casual either. I wanted a ring and I thought he knew it.

I waited. I waited and waited. We'd go to a nice restaurant and I thought, *Oh the ring is in the dessert.* We'd go to the beach, and I thought, *Oh this is a nice place to kneel down.* We went to a friend's wedding, and I thought, well you know what I thought. He asked me once when I was five years old. Come on, do it again. *I won't laugh this time,* I promise. Come on. *GIVE ME THE RING, MOTHERFUCKER!*

Then something extraordinary happened. I met someone. I went on a blind date because my girlfriend needed a fourth, and I met someone when I was most definitely not looking for anyone because my future husband was going to be Mr.

Knightley. So I said I wasn't interested. But the Universe had other plans. We went out to dinner on a Sunday night, and this blind date was really, really cute, and he asked me if he could see me again the next weekend and even though I was not sure if I could live without him, even for the week, I had plans. Mr. Knightley was taking me home to meet his parents. *Oy Vey.*

The weekend with Mr. Knightley and his family went well. I was thoroughly confused and didn't know what to do. On Sunday evening, Mr. Knightley was putting me on the train back to the city. This was it. If he had a ring, I would have put it on. If he had wrapped his arms around me, I would have stayed there forever. If he had just said the word, any word, but especially "Tiffany's" would have worked, my life would have gone in a completely different direction. But instead, he looked into my eyes and said, "Something has changed, hasn't it?"

Was it that obvious?

He took both my hands in his, and he made a small bowl out of them. It was the *Anjali Mudra.* He looked into my eyes and asked if I had met someone. I'm a terrible liar, so I said maybe.

"When you love someone," Mr. Knightley said, "it is like holding a fistful of sand. If you squeeze it too tightly, it will slip through your fingers. If you hold it gently, the sand will stay forever. I am going to let you go, because if you love this man, I cannot keep you. You are not mine to keep. But if he is not the one, and if you come back to me, then, let's make this real."

For the first time in my life, I was clinging to a man. I was desperately hoping this was not happening. This was so Dr.

Zhivago, but at that minute, the train roared into the station and I started to cry. I whined pathetically that I didn't want to go; I wanted to stay with him. I loved him. But he said I had to go and figure it out. I owed it to him, as much as to me. Personal responsibility is a bitch.

I married my blind date six months later. Mr. Knightley knew, even if I didn't.

**You cannot cling to what you do not own.
And in truth, we own nothing.**

Time Is a Great Motivator

How do we let go of the things we love the most and trust that there is more waiting for us? This is the challenge of non-clinging. There has to be something that is a greater motivator than the fear that is holding us back. Of course, there's always time itself.

"Death is very likely the single best invention of life," Steve Jobs told a Stanford audience right after he had been diagnosed with cancer. "It is life's change agent."

Turning fifty means that we do not have all the time left in the world. It makes us take stock of what we want. The spell of mortality, however, is when we are so fixated on the end, or fear of the end, that instead of being motivated to do more, we do less and can become paralyzed in our tracks.

It can go either way. For example, sometimes I tell myself I better try a Handstand now, because tomorrow I will be even older! Or, I can be afraid to try anything new out of fear that I could get hurt. That is clinging to the fear of death. We reach for the things we know will easily bring us success. That is the ego keeping us safe in our zip code. It spins fear like a web and catches us like little flies in its hypnotic trap.

How do we use time as a motivator and break the spell of mortality? How do we let go of the things that do not serve us to make room for new? How do we let go of what we know, for a whole lot of unknown? How can I be good with the Rapture and the possibility of dying today? Even a martini can't completely solve the problem.

The yogi's path is to hold the present lightly, like a fistful of sand. If you can find a kind of acceptance of what is, you'll be able to more skillfully ride the ups and downs. If you can trust that there will always be more, not less, then you will live stronger and more fearless to the end. Instead of having the normal human experience of fear and clinging to a stockpile of memories, you can use the time you have to live fully. You can use time as a change agent, perhaps the greatest change agent of all, to do something now that you have not yet accomplished. It could be that our mortality is not a problem to be solved, but an opportunity to live purposefully while we can. It could be, as Jobs said, the single best invention of life. It is all about how you choose to live.

A Lesson From the Mat

Abundance and Scarcity

There is always more.

If you think otherwise, it is fear. You are clinging to what you have and what you know. The more you cling, the more you will condense what you have, like holding sand. If you squeeze it tightly, the sand will slip through your fingers. If you hold it loosely, it will stay in your hands. But if a great wind comes along and blows all the sand out of your hands anyway, don't worry. There will be more. And it might even be shinier than the last batch.

If you believe in abundance, you will create abundance. That is the lesson of non-clinging.

A Lesson From the Mat

Non-Hoarding, *Aparigraha*

I have a problem with *Aparigraha*. Do you? Be honest.

The *Yoga Sutras* are like the Ten Commandants, Hindu style, and *Aparigraha* is the commandment for non-hoarding, or taking what is truly necessary and no more. The *Sutras* lay down the law for good behavior. Before you can consider yourself a yogi, you must make the effort to live these rules. [See Appendix A.]

I am pretty good with most of them. I am fairly non-violent, although I've been known to throw a dish or two. I can be truthful, when it doesn't involve hurting anyone. I absolutely never steal, unless it's a French fry off my husband's plate. (With his cholesterol, I am doing him a favor by stealing his fries.) I am *uber*-clean and generally lightly perfumed. And I can be extremely content, to the point of being a lazy-ass. But the rule I struggle with the most is *Aparigraha*. B.K.S. Iyengar translated *Aparigraha* as not just having too much stuff, but being without possessions, without belongings, non-acceptance of gifts.

OH MY GOD! You can't accept *gifts?*

My husband says it is critical for me to fully accept *Aparigraha* into my life in order to be a yogi, especially during the Nordstrom Anniversary Sale. I am trying. "Old" Michelle would find a pair of jeans that fit, and buy them in every wash. "New" Michelle only buys one pair, mostly because a yoga teacher has a lot less disposable income than a corporate director. And yet, when my favorite yoga pants go on sale I will buy at least a year's supply in every color. So I guess I have a ways to go before I am a yogi. Life is a paradox, right?

A Lesson From the Mat

The Infinite Game

"There are at least two kinds of games," wrote James Carse in his best-selling book, *The Finite and Infinite Game*. "A finite game is played for the purpose of winning, an infinite game for the purpose of continuing the play."

In life, how do you want to play? When you play to win, there is always a loser. When you play to grow better, you continue to win.

If you attempted a yoga pose and did not succeed, how did you view the practice? Did you lose or did you make progress? If you cling to the outcome of a pose, you are either going to win or lose, but it's harder to practice just to practice. If we can keep our sights on the bigger picture, we can move our practice into the infinite game where we win all the time.

A Lesson From the Mat

Now Is Never

"No man ever steps in the same river twice, for it's not the same river and he's not the same man," said Heraclitus of Ephesus (sometime around 500 BCE).

Yoga teaches us that this moment is all we have and now it is over. And whenever I hear this, I get sad. Really sad. Although it's meant to remind us to make the most of this moment and not let it slip away unnoticed, I can't help feeling that I'm losing something.

This is clinging. I am fearful that the future won't be as good as this moment. In fact, I'm pretty sure it won't be because it will involve making dinner.

However, if we live only for the moment, then we don't have an eye on the future where hope resides. If we live only for the past or the future, then we miss the joys of our present.

Basically, we're screwed either way. Go figure.

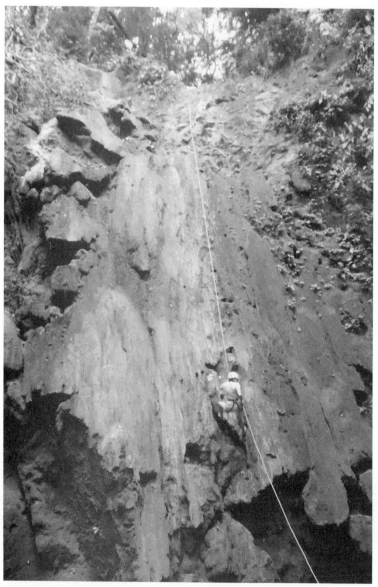
Rock Climbing in Costa Rica. Living yoga off the mat is living more fearlessly.

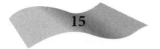

Help Is *Not* on the Way

I am free to take responsibility for my life.
~ Paul Ferrini

I love rock climbing, which is interesting since I am hyper-uncoordinated and phobic about heights.

Of course, I am talking about rock climbing in a gym, where the rocks have nicely spaced little hand- and toe-holds, and a floor filled with spongy doohickeys, and I'm attached to a rope that can swing me like Tarzan. Furthermore, because I am disastrously awkward and terrified, I have a Personal Rock Climbing Coach who stands by me the whole time. When I first started scaling the fifty-foot high wall, I got about halfway up and freaked out.

Me: "Okay, I'm good. How do I get down?"

Personal Rock Climbing Coach: "Are you sure? You are only five feet off the ground."

Me: "Really sure. Please get me down."

PRCC: "Just let go."

Me: "Let go? How?"

PRCC: "Just let go. The rope will catch you."

Me: "I can't let go."

PRCC: "You have to let go."

Me: "I can't let go. And now my fingers have rigor mortis from holding on so tight."

PRCC: "Hmmm. You know what would help?"

Me: "What?"

PRCC: "Yoga. It helps with letting go."

On the second day with the Personal Rock Climbing Coach I arrived early because when you are as much of a klutz as I am, you don't want people to see how long it takes you to put on the harness. Just trying to differentiate the front from the back takes effort. (It's the same with thong underwear, but after a few mistakes, I know now the bigger triangle goes in front. When you don't grow up with computers and thong underwear and a wireless phone, they are all a big mystery.)

I get the rock climbing harness on and attach myself to the wall. I am still early, so I get to thinking: What if this rope thing could hold me up or give me enough support so I can safely do a drop back? A drop back is when you stand up tall in *Tadasana*, Mountain Pose, and you lean way back into *Urdvha Dhanurasana*, Wheel, so your hands reach the floor. I decide to go for it.

I stand up tall, lift my heart to the sky, lean waaaaaayyy back, and fall on my head.

"Oh my God!" I scream in shock and not a little bit of pain.

Everybody turns and stares at the crazy woman on the floor covered in spongy doohickeys. I assure them I'm okay, but my Personal Rock Climbing Coach gets in trouble, because one of the reasons he was assigned to me is that totally uncoordinated people should not be left alone even for a minute with rock climbing equipment. They may think they are more capable than they truly are.

What Holds You Back?

Two months after the disastrous attempted drop back with the rock climbing equipment, I did a drop back for the first time on my own. I was at a yoga workshop in Tucson where we had partners to help take us back. The trick in taking someone backwards to the floor is to know just how much help they need. Sometimes you need to offer a firm hold and sometimes not.

I was in the second camp, where I'd been doing this so long it's slightly ridiculous that I'm still afraid to drop back unassisted. I have a stronger backbend than ever; I know the yoga principles involved; I am just a chicken shit. So I told my partner to be there just in case. But instead, she gave me the full-Nelson wrap-around hip lock. The second time, I again asked, nicely, for just a little support, and again she gave me the full hold. The third time, again, big full-supported hold. Then I got pissed off. And on my fourth time dropping back I pushed her away and went for it. *Ta da!*

If I was going to do it, I would need to do it by myself.

"Help is *not* on the way," Baron Baptiste said during a one-day Immersion in Denver in 2009. "What is holding you back?" he said. "You need to ask yourself this question every day: Why am I not achieving the things I said I would? Why?"

As soon as I fully grasped that no one would, or could, save me, I was free to save myself.

What If You Had No Problems?

Can you even imagine if you had no problems?

I remember the moment I first considered the possibility. Desiree Rumbaugh suggested that perhaps it was as easy as saying so. Maybe having no problems is just about shifting your perspective.

And suddenly, it was as if I had no problems. I realized that most of my problems were in my head.

I don't want to belittle the trials and tribulations of life. Life can be very hard. People can be a pain in the rear. We can have illness and financial worries. Our children may suffer. We might fall on our face and fail. But having a problem on the outside is different from making it a problem on the inside. We have very little control of how fate is going to roll the dice. But we have a lot of control determining how we are going to react to it.

Good Luck, Bad Luck!

There is a Chinese proverb about luck that speaks to whether or not we have problems. Once upon a time there was a farmer whose horse ran away. When the neighbors said, "What bad luck," the farmer replied, "Bad luck? Good luck? Who knows?"

A week later, the horse returned with a herd of horses from the hills. Now the neighbors said, "What good luck." His answer was, "Good luck? Bad luck? Who knows?"

Then the farmer's son broke his leg while trying to tame the wild horses. Everyone thought this was very bad luck. But the farmer said, "Bad luck? Good luck? Who knows?"

Some weeks later, the army marched into the village and enlisted all the young men. When they saw the farmer's son with his broken leg, they left him alone. Good luck? Bad Luck? Who knows?

This parable is one reason why I don't necessarily believe in luck. We don't have the luxury of knowing how the future will turn out. Things that seem to be problems may turn out to be good fortune instead.

**It is just as easy to believe
that the Universe is conspiring *for* us,
rather than against us.**

Although I am from New York and was raised in a "sky is falling" mentality, this is the biggest transformation in my life since I started practicing yoga. Now I root myself in the concept that I don't really have any problems. I practice gratitude. When I start to fear the future, I get on my mat. And when shit happens, I say, "Of course!" Good luck? Bad luck? Who knows?

Yet even wizened old yogis have lapses where we are quick to believe what we want to believe. An astrologer told me once that a particular year was going to be huge, HUGE, for me. I completely forgot my rule of good luck, bad luck, who knows. Instead, I jumped for joy. Then almost immediately, the "huge year" happened. First my son tore the ACL in his knee. Then my father-in-law, whom I loved dearly, passed away, and then my beloved dog passed away, and then the IRS audited us, and then my mother was diagnosed with a fast growing cancer, and then, and then, and then...

When I look back on that year, the good news was that my son became a straight A student. And although life tried to pull me further off course from the work I loved, I buckled down more relentlessly than ever before and found success.

One thing I learned:

**Problems don't go away,
but we can learn how to navigate them more skillfully.**

Ganesha Is My Om-Boy

Ganesha is the elephant-headed Hindu deity, the remover of obstacles. We pray to him not because Ganesha's life was easy, but because he always found solutions. Take his head, for instance. His mother could not conceive a baby (problem) so she created Ganesha out of the dust on her skin (solution). Then one day she asked him to guard her while she took a bath. He was doing a great job until his father, Lord Shiva, who had never seen his son, came home. Shiva did not like being barred from Parvati (problem), so he cut off Ganesha's head (solution). Parvati was furious (problem) and told Shiva to fix this right away. Shiva looked for a head and the first animal he saw was the mighty elephant, so he chopped off the beast's head and gave it to his son (solution). Ganesha became mightier than ever.

Later, when Ganesha grew up, he was a witness to the battle described in the epic poem the *Bhagavad Gita*. At the time, he thought the story should be documented but he did not have a pen. So he broke off his tusk, dipped it into the river of blood from the fallen warriors and wrote down what he saw. Problem solved.

The heroes among us are never the ones who had it easy. They are the people who faced great personal challenges, yet used their problems to become better, to transform themselves. They didn't wait for help. They did it now.

Atha, Now

Atha is the first word of the *Yoga Sutras*. It means, "Now." Yoga doesn't begin when we have time, when all the problems go away, when we have a free afternoon to meditate.

Yoga begins now.

Now, we get to live our life. Now, we get to be better people. Now, we get to work out our problems. Not later, now.

Contrary to what some believe, you don't have to take a year off of your life so you can hang out in an ashram. Yoga begins now, when you have lost your job and nobody else is stepping up to pay your rent; when you have done wrong and you feel terrible; when you are in pain; when you have problems. *Atha*.

As a yoga teacher, I am never quite as fascinated by those who can effortlessly slide into poses. I am more interested in the rest of us who struggle. When the road gets tough, that's when it gets useful.

Get Out of Your Way

"The only thing standing between me and greatness is me," said Woody Allen.

I'm in the same boat. I need to get out of my own way, especially on the yoga mat. To live a problem-free life, I need to start with my mind. The mind is the greatest problem maker I have. Of the mind, body and spirit, the mind pipes up the most with all the reasons why I won't be successful. The mind is often saying, "Uh oh." In fact, my mind says *you suck; you look ridiculous in those yoga pants; and what is up with that hair?* To live a problem-free life, I need to get the mind to be on my team, and I need to stop defining myself by my problems.

I invite you to consider:

- Anatomy is not destiny. Your arms are not too short. Your legs are not too long. Your butt is not too heavy. Your body is fine.
- You are what you say you are. If you say, "I am not strong," then you create that reality. Same with, "I am not flexible."
- You can be anything you want to be, and if you say it out loud, you might start to believe it. More importantly, if you say it to someone else, they might believe it and encourage you to continue. And if you write it on Facebook, then it will definitely come true.

Furthermore, it is very important to let go of what does not serve us, like when we realize that certain people in our life are not doing us any good. The mind is a frenemy, not entirely a friend, not entirely an enemy. It's just a friend we need to watch carefully in case it tries to steal our self-confidence the way a frenemy would steal a boyfriend.

Things to know about the mind:
- It is a frenemy. Be cautious when it tells you something.
- It is a problem-making machine. We attach to comments made *about* us, *by* us and *to* us. We can make mountains out of molehills. We are all, generally, a little crazy.
- Just as easily as it can attach, the mind can also detach. We can take a "witness consciousness," where we can be objective and think, *Here is a problem, now what can be done about it,* rather than, *"OMG, this is all about MEEEEEEEEEE!"*

Own It

Part of solving problems, of living a problem-free life, is to stand up and own them in the first place. You cannot fix anything if you don't first take responsibility. If you don't own it, you can't fix it.

"You can take responsibility at any time," a teacher once told me. It's so simple, and true.

I have a girlfriend who went through a divorce. While she did all the usual things to get over it, the change did not come for her until she owned her part in the situation. It was easy to blame her ex for everything. (Actually, we all blame him as well.) But once she took responsibility, she could move on. "When I owned it, I could let it go," she said.

Taking responsibility is a bitch, but it's at the heart of living a problem-free life. It is easier to wallow in your misery and cry poor, poor me than to stand up and be a warrior. It is easier to blame everyone else, than to say, I had a part in this. It is easier to regret the past, than searching out your own shortcomings and actually changing them. But the easier path is not always the better path. It's like relying on a rock-climbing harness to drop you back, when in reality, you will only get dropped on your head, over and over again.

I find it interesting that I have a much easier time finding my balance in Handstand when I don't have help, than when someone is there holding my leg. When I have a crutch, I need it. When I am forced to do it on my own, I rise up and balance. When my teenage son started to drive, I told him I was very nervous about certain things he still did when I was in the car. "But Mom, you don't understand," he said. "When I'm on my own, I'll be more careful because I'll be on my own."

I totally get it. He knows that help is not right there, so he will be more alert, more careful and more conscientious. He will own it. It is the same for all of us. When we realize we are free, at any time, to take responsibility for our lives, we live the life we were meant to live. Or, we can wait for help and hope it's on the way.

Just don't count on the rock climbing rope to hold you up if you try a drop back. I learned it's better to do it on your own.

A Lesson From the Mat

About Control

Three things you cannot control (so stop trying):

1. Life: It's not fair.
2. People: They will let you down.
3. Actions: Things do not always turn out the way you think, but the way things turn out could be better than you originally thought.

Things you CAN change (so start trying):

1. Your mind.
2. Your attitude.
3. Your health.
4. How you recognize the gifts in your life. Be grateful.
5. Your friends. Spend time with people you admire and let go of those who do not serve you in a way that's life affirming. Unless they are family; then you are kind of stuck with them.
6. Quit whining.
7. Realize you are free to take responsibility at any time.

A Lesson From the Mat

The *Kleshas*, Afflictions in Life

- Ignorance
- Ego (or too much pride)
- Attachment to pleasure
- Aversion to pain
- Fear of death (or clinging to life)

Notice that the afflictions that hold us back, that keep us from being our strongest self, that make our yoga practice weak on the mat, and make us a bunch of whiners off the mat, have nothing to do with our physical bodies. Rather, the *kleshas* dwell in the space between our ears.

A Lesson From the Mat

The *Malas*, Temporary Problems or Veils

The *Malas* hide our true self-worth from us. They afflict each of us now and then.

- *Anava Mala:* Feelings of unworthiness, shame, disgrace, sadness and depression.
- *Mayiya Mala*: Feelings of separation, isolation, conflict, and anger.
- *Karma Mala*: Feelings of anxiety, fear and doer-ship (feeling like you need to get more done).

The *Malas* are problems, true, yet we can use them to make ourselves better. So if you feel unworthy, try helping someone else. If you feel isolated, pick up the phone and call a friend. If you feel like you need to get more done, try doing less! This is how our "problems" can become a practice instead.

A Lesson From the Mat

What You Can Do

Look Ma! Look what I can do!

Sometimes when I'm on my mat, it seems like everyone around me is moving gracefully or holding their poses without effort, and I'm in Child's Pose, *Balasana*. Of course, it may be because I'm tired that day, or twenty years older than everyone else. But whatever, it's easy to think, "I can't."

I know the meaning of "I can't." When I was fifteen, my mother was diagnosed with Multiple Sclerosis, which meant she would be in and out of wheelchairs for the rest of her life. I was radically aware of what "can't" meant: she can't walk, can't talk, can't be Mom the way she used to be. There are times you must take care of yourself. That is being a responsible adult. But then there are also times you give up.

It is just as easy to think, I can, rather than I can't.

When I come to my mat, especially on the days when I don't feel like it or when I am tired, I usually have a lovely practice. Instead of thinking "I can't," yoga has shown me how to look for the "I can" along the way. When I see a pose that is currently impossible for me, I look for the possibility in it. I look for what I *can* do.

There is always some part of it that I can attempt. These are the building blocks to a stronger practice. Quitting never gets you very far. Saying, "Look what I can do," will get you farther.

Passion, Practice and Presence

Practice means to perform,
over and over again in the face of all obstacles,
some act of vision, of faith, of desire.
Practice is a means of inviting the perfection desired.
~ Martha Graham

To age gracefully is to not become obsolete. To age gracefully is to become more proficient, more practiced and more present with the things you love. I believe, in the end, it is passion that keeps us going.

For my grandfather, Sam Berman, his passion was his work. Sam wouldn't mind if he had died at his desk, and he very nearly did. He tried retirement for one day. Then he looked around his empty apartment (my grandmother had passed on by then), and went back to work. He took vacations, enjoyed the opera, attended synagogue, but come Monday you could count on him being back at his desk where he hoped to make a difference for the company he loved.

"I'll be here until they carry me out, toes up," he liked to say.

I've come to realize that for him, work was more than just a paycheck and something to do or a place to go. His company was his passion.

Passion is one secret to living stronger.

Passion is the nectar on which we thrive. Every person who I find inspiring has something in their lives that keeps them motivated and interested. My stepmother loves to cook and has studied with many world famous chefs. Her dinner parties are legendary. When we talk on the holidays, she always asks what I made for dinner. (Um, reservations?) I have another girlfriend who discovered tennis later in life, and now she travels like a teenager to tournaments. My mother turned sixty-five and discovered that the state of Florida offers senior citizens huge discounts to audit university classes. Did you know that instead of reversing the loss of brain cells brought on by young children, teenagers and long life, you can actually "exercise" them back to good health? So my Mom decided that retirement might be a great time to get another PhD, this time in biological statistics. Of course it is!

Every interesting person I know has something to be crazy about. For me, it is standing on my head.

Passion Keeps Us Young

Before there was yoga to fill my every waking moment, there were horses. I was a passionate rider. From the time I was five years old, I rode. I went to riding camps in the summer, and started to ride in official shows when I was six. My little feet could barely reach the stirrups, but I would trot around the ring with a smile so big that it could light up a judge, and often did.

Even though my family could not quite afford one of the world's most expensive pastimes, it did not stop me. As a teenager I earned my riding lessons by spending my summers working in a stable tending the horses for the Hamptons' rich and famous. My dream then was to make it to the biggest A-rated show in the country held at Madison Square Garden. Sometimes after work, we'd grab the horses from the fields and take them out for a ride with nothing more than two lead lines attached to a halter. Bareback and barefoot, we'd go careening down the silver sands of Long Island's beaches, then head into the nearby potato fields to race among the rows of the leafy greens. I remember those days like yesterday.

I chose my college because it had an equestrian team. Seriously. Forget that it had a renowned English department, or the state's best nursing school. I went for the horses. When people ask if I had a sport in college, I can say, "Yes, I rode." But it turned out to be brief, since the sport required a financial commitment I just could not maintain. Not to mention upholding my grades!

Later, I worked in several careers but I never gave up my passion. As a journalist in Alabama, I found a farm that needed riders and learned how to train racehorses. There is nothing in the world like being the first person ever to get on top of a young, green horse. Exhilarating does not come close to describing it. While some cowboys would use strength to control the horse, I chose love, and usually the horse responded well. However, there were plenty of times that I ended up in the dirt.

I rode almost every day of my life until I was pregnant with my first son. And just like that, the thing I loved the most was not as important as the little person inside me I had not yet met. So I quit. I stopped riding for two babies, preschool, and kindergarten—all told about seven years. Then when my youngest went to school full time, I went back to riding and promptly hurt my back. Although I felt the same, apparently things were not the same in me at all. (Really, one good look in the mirror would have told me that.) I was older, weaker, and distracted by motherhood.

When I look back to the time when I lost my ability to ride, I was utterly lost, like a ship without a rudder. I had no driving passion in my life except for children and family. I was truly at a complete loss without my own interests to follow. And I was very aware that if you put everything into your children and if you do it very well, then someday they will leave you. That sucks.

"It does not matter what you do when you grow up," my grandfather Raphael Weissman used to say, "As long as you do it well, and be the best you can be. If you are a housekeeper, then be the best housekeeper, and you will have pride in your work."

It is so interesting to me that my love for horses is what brought me to yoga. It was the Universe's Plan B for my life. If I had not gone back to riding and hurt myself, if I did not want to ride again so obsessively that I was willing to suffer through physical therapy and Pilates to get stronger, then I would never have found my mat.

Does anything random truly happen in life?

Yoga was meant to heal my back, but instead became the all-consuming passion that I needed to save my life after riding became impossible. It became the thing in my life that has kept me young and strong, and most of all, interesting. Yoga is my fearless heart, in action.

Invite More In — Practice

Practice is the invitation to more. If passion is our fearless heart in action, then practice is the steady perseverance we need to show up. Practice is the way we express our devotion, and how we invite more into our lives.

"Eighty percent of success is showing up," said Woody Allen. Some days, it is all I can do to haul my tired butt to the mat, but somewhere around my twentieth Downward Facing Dog, *Adho Mukha Svanasana,* I am glad I did. Practice is devotion in motion. Practice will keep you focused, challenged, and on the path. Practice will also keep life in perspective.

My first yoga practice was based on Ashtanga Yoga. It is a series of repetitive movements, performed over and over again, from the primary through advanced sequences. There is something extremely comforting in repetitious movements, the way a Catholic recites the rosary or a Muslim bows down to the Ka'aba in Mecca in prayer.

In Ashtanga, you tie together breath and movement, what some call a "moving meditation." In the Mysore version of the practice, people come together to practice individually, but the sequences they perform are the same. The same, yet different. We are connected to each other through breath and the series of postures, but we maintain our individuality.

Although I loved the repetition of Ashtanga, in the end my shoulders gave out. I was also stuck in the primary levels for a long time. From Ashtanga, I went to Power/Vinyasa. In the Vinyasa practice, the moves are based on Ashtanga, but you can dance around like the Sugarplum Fairy. (Although I looked like I'd had a few more sugarplums than the average fairy.) Now I practice align and flow formats. So you are free to find more advanced poses as you learn along the way. And I try a little Hot Yoga, too sometimes.

It does not matter which type of yoga you practice. The best yoga is the one you do. Practice and studentship, or *adikara*, is the quality we want to cultivate. The more we show up on our mats, the more we are able to look inward and discover more. This in turn, creates increased focus and increased dedication. It is Presence.

Be Present

Of course, the most passionate and the most devoted student who comes to the mat to practice every day, must still put the lessons he learns into action. And that would be through Presence.

Presence is the reward of yoga.

If I could change one thing about myself, it would be having the ability to maintain more presence in the moment. I'd like to be here, not "there," for my family and friends. I'd like to be fully vested in the now. But instead, I'm often running around, working, making dinner (*Yes, sometimes.*) driving carpool, rushing to teach, rushing to practice, rushing, rushing, and rushing. If I'm not multi-tasking, I feel like I'm slacking off. Just the other day, I was speaking to a friend on the phone while folding laundry. Then I packed my yoga bag and left to practice. I was halfway to the studio before I realized I hadn't heard a thing she said.

I'm sure I'm not the only one who struggles with the now. Eve might not have been paying attention when she got those instructions about the apple. Even the Warrior Arjuna in the *Bhagavad Gita* struggled with it, worrying about the future and the past as a way to escape what he must do in the present. So apparently, it's been a problem for thousands of years.

Yet when I think about the people in my life who have meant so much to me, it is those who gave me their fullest attention: a college professor who had faith in me, or a girlfriend who wholeheartedly listened. Now and then my father or mother will call on the phone, and I know they are absolutely "there" in the conversation. My grandfather Sam had this ability when he focused on you, for you to believe there was nothing else in the world that mattered. People say that when you spoke to Jacqueline Kennedy Onassis, she had a way of focusing her attention so you felt you were the most fascinating thing to her on the earth at that moment.

I want to be like that for the ones I love. I want my family and friends to know I am completely there for them. I want my students to know I am paying attention. But most of all, I want to be completely there for me. Showing up is my secret desire. I wish to be there, fully, wherever I am, and I believe that practicing this passion will invite more presence into my life.

A Lesson From the Mat

Show Up!

It's easy to spot the students in class who are not really there. One clue is they are whispering to friends or texting on their cell phones. Another clue is they are busy doing their own practice. Or they might be sitting with their eyes closed because whatever is in their head is far more interesting than what the yoga teacher has to say.

I tend to ignore the students who show up, but who *do not show up* for class. After all, there are many others who are looking to build a stronger practice who benefit from my instruction. Ironically, the students who are not present, do not get as much attention or refinement to their practice, and so they may further withdraw and do their own thing. As a teacher, I try to reverse this *samskara*, or the rut caused by the stupid things we do, by focusing on the students who are *not* there. But really, it's ridiculous. Like the adults in the Peanuts cartoon, this is how I sound to them: "Waa, waaa, waaaaa."

In the end, you have to make the decision: How do you want to practice? Do you want to show up? How much do you want to be present? If you can show up on your mat, chances are you can do this in the rest of your life as well.

A Lesson From the Mat

How Much Do You Want It?

You may have to ask yourself, do you really want this thing, this skill or this new obsession? If so, go for it. That is Passion.

What are you willing to do for it? Are you willing to try? Are you willing to practice?

Practice is the investment you make in your dreams. When people tell me they would like to be able to do a certain yoga pose, I tell them anything is within reach but they will need to practice it at least twice a day. They look at me like I'm crazy. I'm not crazy; I'm committed.

Don't let anyone or anything take you away from your dreams. That is the focus you'll need to get it done.

A Lesson From the Mat

Be Creative

If you create something, then it's a chance to stay vital in life.

As we age, our time is often taken up with the nuts and bolts of existence like paying the bills and taking care of our family. The time we have to create something new or artistic is limited.

Yet this is one thing I believe: that if you find an outlet for creative energy, you will feel more connected to the world. If you contribute something, whether it is artistic or simply an expression of a deeper understanding about life, then you remain relevant. You create positive energy, your mind is stimulated and you enhance your sense of well being and personal growth.

My yoga practice is an opportunity to create an artistic offering in a pose. I also enjoy painting, decorating and will someday have more time to play with my camera. My mother loves photography as well as painting, and when she lived in Okinawa with my father, she learned how to do a variety of Japanese arts.

Some may like to draw, others sing. A few spend their time creating the perfect fishing fly out of minute filament.

Once, my son dropped an extra-curricular course on computers to take a course on art. I was thrilled.

"I saw the angel in the marble and carved until I set him free," explained Michelangelo. But the truth is, the one who is set free is the creator.

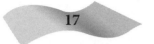

Choose!

Nothing has a stronger influence...on their children,
than the unlived lives of the parents.
~ Carl Jung

It was a turtle that led me to yoga.

What does it mean to become a yogi? Is it when you discover your mat? Or is it when you wake up and live a more conscious life? Or could it be when you realize your *dharma*, your duty? I believe it is all those things, and one more: I believe it is when you choose.

I first had to choose whether to look the other way or to stand up for a moral code that I did not yet know was a part of me, when I was just ten years old. I was all legs, arms, and freckles, and at the height of pre-teen awkwardness. By then, I had little memory of my parents ever having been together, and my Dad was something of a mystery as well. I lived with my mother and grandmother, and various other women who rode in and out of our lives: some on motorcycles, some in VW campers, and some on the bus. Women, I understood. Men, not so much.

My parents had now been divorced for twice as long as they were married, and I saw my father once a month, which often left me wanting more. At ten, I was full of questions and very few answers.

It was a time of unease in our lives. My Mom was deep into finding herself, and was moving us around from one adventure to the next. I had missed more school than a kid in a circus. We traveled with theater companies, lived on a boat, and even spent time in the Blue Ridge Mountains, wherever they are.

My Dad was worried. But he too was unsettled. Truthfully, there are some men who just do better being married than on their own, even if it's to the wrong woman. I think it was dawning on him that his second marriage was on the rocks as well.

So we did what many people do when things are confusing. We decided to get as far away from our troubles as we could get. In our case, Dad chose a luxury resort in the British Virgin Islands for he and his wife (my stepmother), and me. If you are confused and miserable, then by all means grab a preteen adolescent for your vacation. I was overjoyed.

We stayed in a cottage surrounded by pink and yellow flowers with a view of the ocean that stretched forever. The resort was shaped like a crescent moon, with our bungalow at one end on top of a hill, and the resort at the other. In the middle the beach stretched its pink sands like the soft underbelly of a sleeping cat. At night you listened to the waves lapping the shore.

I had a room to myself. I remember my bed being up against a wall with a large window where I could watch the sea. At first, I was excited to have my own room. But I quickly realized that having a friend along would have been really nice. In fact, that was my childhood theme: with all that moving around a friend would have been really nice. To compensate, I made one up. Her name was "Karen" and I brought her with me wherever I went. I decided it might be time to take Karen out to play.

At breakfast, my father and stepmother enrolled me in the Kid's Club, which would take up every spare minute of the day, and if there had been a Kid's Club at night, they would have put me in that as well. I knew a losing battle when I saw one, so I happily trotted off, yet walked out again by lunch. Nobody had to know. I just took Karen by the hand and did my own thing. I went up to the cottage and curled up with a book.

At dinner, we made small talk and my Dad asked about camp and I said, "It's fine." The waiter came over and detailed the evening's offerings, including the specialty of the house, which was the turtle soup. This resort was known for its turtle soup. It was world famous.

"What makes the soup so good?" my father asked.

"We use our own turtles," the waiter replied.

We three sat speechless.

What the what! There are turtles in turtle soup? I thought it was chicken; every other weird thing in the world was usually just chicken, like the Halloween Green Guts Goulash, it was just chicken and vegetables with food coloring. And chocolate "turtles" are caramel and nuts. Welsh rarebit doesn't have any baby rabbit in it. So what is up with the turtle soup?

I had always been a little queasy about eating meat, except for chickens, which if you've ever spent a lot of time around chickens, you would know it might be okay to eat them. Baby chicks, not so much. You can pet a baby chick. However, big grown, squawking chickens, *ewwwww.*

But turtles? Come on. These are magnificent creatures. They live for a long time. Their steadfastness beats the hare's speed. In Hinduism, there is a story about how Lord Vishnu saves the world from a flood by becoming Kurma, a huge turtle and allowing the last mountain to float on his back. *A turtle saves the world! And now I'm supposed to eat one in a bowl of soup?*

I could see Dad blanch, yet ever the gentleman, he said nothing. He ordered something else. I stuck my finger down my throat and made retching noises while my stepmother complained about "the child" again. It was just another family dinner.

Afterwards, my father held my hand for a walk and we meandered down the beach all the way to our cottage at the end of the property. It felt so good to be in his grip. Dad has great hands; they are the skilled hands of a surgeon, strong, able and adept. I adored him, even if he was something of a stranger to me. My stepmother opted out when we got to the cottage, so Dad and I continued alone on the path until we found ourselves at a labyrinth of stone walls on the beach.

I jumped on top of the nearest rock and started tiptoeing along the wall pretending to be a gymnast on a beam. I was trying not to fall, when I saw something splash. Then I saw a flipper, and when I bent down closer, I saw his face.

"Dad," I screeched. "There are turtles in here!"

He quickly came by my side. We sat on the stone wall and watched those turtles swim in their pen for at least half an hour. There were babies, and a lot of medium sized turtles, and one humongous one. "Is that one a grandpa?" I asked him.

"I don't know," he said, "But turtles are magnificent. They live for hundreds of years. Nobody has the right to cage a turtle. They are the kings of the sea."

We sat quietly. I was fighting back the tears as I realized these turtles would be soup the next day. And so, before either of us knew it, we had hatched a plan.

We had to choose between the rules and what was right. We chose the turtles.

Dad waded into the pen and started lifting out the turtles, one by one. I jumped in but the turtles were big—much bigger than I—so I could only heave the babies to freedom. We freed about a half dozen before it was too dark to see their shadowy shapes in the water.

The next night, after dinner, we went back to the pen. This time we worked quickly and precisely. Dad told me to stand on the wall and watch for people. He jumped into the pen and one by one, set the turtles free. He'd chase one around and back it into a corner, then grab its massive shell and fling it over the edge. I could have sworn that once the turtles figured out what we were up to, they began to swim to us. He was able to throw at least nine turtles over the rock wall before it became too dark.

We returned the next night. By now, most of the smaller ones were gone and only the larger, heavier ones remained, and the giant "grandpa" turtle. He looked extremely sad to me, as if he knew he was just too big to get over the wall. Dad was worried we had thinned out the group so much that the hotel would become suspicious. He said the hotel most likely wouldn't kill the smaller ones for quite a while because they wouldn't provide enough meat. And the big grandpa was just too big for him to lift by himself. So I started to cry. Like most men, my Dad cannot stand crying. It kills him.

At dinner the following night, my father asked the waiter for the day's specials. The waiter recited a few things, but no turtle soup.

"No turtle soup?" my father asked, giving me a wink. "Why not? Have the turtles left the island?"

When we went down to the pen that evening it had been marked off with yellow tape, and large "Do Not Trespass" signs were posted. In addition, there was a sign that anyone caught poaching the turtles would be fined and there could be imprisonment. My Dad weighed this carefully and decided that ending the vacation in jail was not the bonding experience he had in mind.

"But what about the grandpa?" I whined.

"He's lived several hundred years, sweetheart. I'm sure he'll figure out a way to live a few more."

But I wasn't so sure. The next day, I moped around the hotel room. It was our last day at the resort, and I was miserable. At dinner, my father couldn't take it anymore.

"All right," he said. "We'll try to set him free."

To choose is not always easy.

A choice is not often between the obvious right and wrong. There may not be anyone else on your side. You may even end up in jail. But you know you have done the right thing when you cannot live with yourself having done anything else. That night, we chose the turtles over the law.

We had to wait until it got a little darker than usual, and then we crept down to the stone walls and waited. Dad said I was to be the lookout as he waded into the pen. The massive turtle came right up to him, but my father could not lift him up.

"If we're going to do this," he said, "I'll need help."

So I jumped in the water and grabbed hold of the turtle's shell. Wow, was he heavy. We heaved, and nothing. Instead of lifting him over the middle of the wall where it was highest, we decided to coax the turtle to the sandy edge of the pen where the wall was barely a foot tall. He swam willingly. Then with Dad at the front, and me at the back, we somehow managed to boost him up to the top of the wall, and gently scraped his belly over the pen.

The turtle tumbled into the sandy shallow water and then floated still as if in shock. I was afraid he was hurt from the rock wall scraping his belly. But instead, he seemed to turn and gaze at us. I looked directly into his wise old eyes and I thought he said thank you. Then with a blink of his heavy lids, he turned and moved surprisingly fast toward the open sea. In a few seconds, he was gone.

Yoga Is Choice

When does yoga begin? The *Yoga Sutras* tell us it is *atha*, "now." Yoga begins now, and now is when you choose.

I became a yogi at ten. I would be fifty years old before I understood what it meant and how to step into the power of action. But at that moment, guided by my father, I realized that there was only one path we could take. It was our *dharma*, our duty at the time.

**As humans, we are given the gift of choice.
It is a powerful gift.**

We must choose what to believe in. We must choose who we love. We must choose when to fight and when to lay down our sword. The Gods and Goddesses of Hindu literature have a more limited existence as they do not always have the full gamut of choice; Hanuman's *dharma* is to serve, Vishnu's *dharma* to lead, Lakshmi's *dharma* is to be rich and beautiful. (It's tough, but someone has to do it.) We, on the other hand, can choose our path.

Yoga is only a little bit about the postures. The postures are useful to reveal who we are and how we react when things get difficult. Our yoga practice is a constant practice of choice. How we live on the mat is endlessly revealing about how we live off the mat. Yoga is ultimately about discovering ourselves on the mat, and taking that knowledge into service in our lives.

I realized that the moment I looked into that turtle's eyes, I became awake to my sense of right and wrong, to my sense of duty. He was my teacher. I could see the injustice of caging him to die. Of course, neither of us had heard of yoga in

1970. But yoga is not just the poses you can see, but also it's about the part of the world you cannot see.

"There is a field between right and wrong," said the poet Rumi. "I will meet you there." In the field of right and wrong is the path of choice. This is where we set our mat. Yoga is about leaving the world a better place and finding our path in the field. In that moment, so many years ago, there was no question about what we would do. The choice was clear.

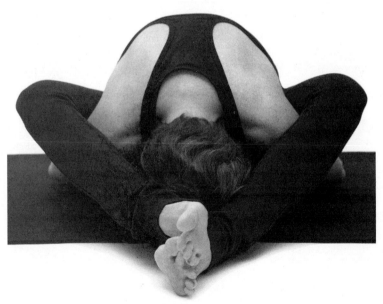

Tortoise Pose, *Kurmasana*, named for Lord Kurma who saved the world.

A Lesson From the Mat

When You Choose Badly: *Samskaras*

Humans have a knack for accumulating *samskaras*, which are the stupid things we do. Like a girlfriend who always chooses the wrong kind of guy. Or doing the same thing over and over again, like saying we are not flexible, or cannot do a Handstand. Or we have the same arguments with someone when we know there is no "winning." (This might explain some of those pesky family relationships; they are *samskaras*.)

Our *samskaras* live way below the surface of our consciousness.

Although it is easier to see all the unconscious stuff everyone else does, it is nearly impossible to have this vision with ourselves. This in turn, affects our *karma*.

To make better decisions, we must see our *samskaras* by bringing them up from the deep into the light. If you get a glimpse, if someone tells you, for example, about the dimwitted things you do, don't run away. Embrace it as a chance to do better and change. Choosing to see all of you is choosing more in your life.

A Lesson From the Mat

Clean Your Karma

Don't worry. If you made a bad decision, there's always Kali.

There are three main Goddesses in the Hindu tradition: Saraswati, Lakshmi and Kali. Saraswati, the Goddess of wisdom, brings culture and refinement to the world. Lakshmi is the Goddess of beauty, wealth and happiness. Then there is Kali. Kali brings about transformation.

Kali is, for lack of a better word, a very competent bitch. One day there was a huge battle on earth and the people ran to Lord Shiva for help. He was busy meditating, of course, so he asked his wife, Parvati to take care of it. Parvati was not going to do battle with a thousand multi-headed demons, so she created Kali, the "Black One," a ferocious fighter. Kali defeated the demons, although she went a little crazy. To stop her rampage, Shiva ran down from the mountain to lie down at Kali's feet. When she recognized him, she put down her sword.

Not surprisingly, Kali is also known for motherly love. If this makes no sense, try pissing off a mother lion and see how far you get.

Of the three Goddesses, Kali is the one powerful enough to clean *karma*, the cycle of cause and effect created by our actions. *Karma* is very powerful, but Kali is more powerful.

So if you have chosen badly, then pray to Kali, and be a relentless warrior in cleaning up your life. Kali welcomes any and all battles; nothing is too great for her. It is never too late to cleanse your *karma*, but you need to go Kali on it. You need to be ferociously *good* and your *karma* will change.

A Lesson From the Mat

Choose the Divine

At the heart of the *Bhagavad Gita*, an epic poem written down in the fifth century, is the question of choice. To choose is the first step of yoga.

The story takes place on a battlefield. Arjuna, the greatest living warrior of all time is preparing to do battle. He pulls up to the field, but instead of getting ready to fight, he puts down his sword. He realizes that among the warriors on the other side are his family and friends. He is deeply torn and doesn't know what to do. The battlefield becomes a symbol of the battles we face, within and without.

Arjuna is offered a choice. He can choose the army, or he can choose Krishna. He chooses the Divine. Then, in the following eighteen chapters, Krishna guides him to make the second biggest decision of his life, whether or not to fight. Ultimately the choice is his.

"I have no more doubts," he tells Krishna at the end. "I will act according to your command." Accepting his *dharma*, his duty, and knowing that he will act in accordance with God, is everything to Arjuna. Acting according to the moral compass is that which we seek. To choose is to live our yoga.

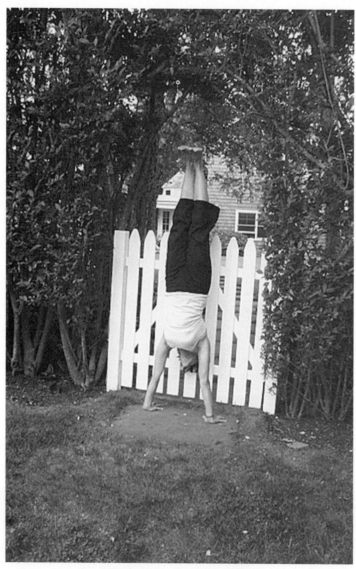

Pose: Handstand, *Adho Mukha Vrksasana.*
Home again, home again, jiggity jig.

18

Arrive!

If we tidy and clean our house enough,
we might notice that divinity has been sitting in it all along.
~ B.K.S. Iyengar

It's never too late to write a new ending for your story.

The story of our life, the one with the white picket fence, seldom turns out as we expected. But, I offer this: it could be better.

My father, for example, did not intend to be a famous small animal veterinarian in New York City. Rather, he dreamed of escaping the city. He wanted to be a gentleman farmer and have a little acreage in Vermont. At sixteen, he was accepted to Cornell University, enrolled at the College of Agricultural, and prepared for his exodus by studying everything he'd need to know to be a farmer.

Then the day came when he needed to check a cow's ovaries for insemination. And guess what? His arms were too short.

"Lewis," his teacher said upon seeing Dad buried up to the armpit in this cow, "You are going to have to change your plans." That is how the world got, what *Vogue* called the "Jet Set Pet Vet." He became one of the greatest veterinarians to treat small animals. It was Plan B.

Plan B Is the Universe's Plan

Rule number one: When shit happens, these moments are often the turning points in life.

When I was fifteen, my only plan was to have fun. I was a sophomore in a very small boarding school tucked away in the Berkshire Mountains. We were smart, we were somewhat privileged, and like teenagers everywhere, we assumed the world was ours. I was busy playing soccer in the fall, skiing in the winter, and sunbathing amongst the lilacs in the spring. I had all the time in the world and nothing more on my mind than what to wear on Saturday night. Then the phone rang. My mother was in the hospital and I needed to go home.

Back in New York, Mom was reaching the final conclusion of a health odyssey that began when she was in her twenties. She was frequently in and out of hospitals. She had been told over the years that she had cancer, leukemia, polio, and that she was just plain crazy. Now crazy had a name: Multiple Sclerosis. She would spend the rest of her life in and out of wheelchairs and hospitals.

After moving eighteen times and going to six different schools, I had hoped to finish high school in this one place I had come to call home. Now suddenly, the odds of my being able to finish did not look so good. Mom needed help, so at fifteen, I became the mom to Mom.

I spent that early spring taking care of her in the hospital, bathing her, washing her hair, seeing that the doctors were paying attention. Her recovery was slow. Then someone remembered that I should be in school. I think perhaps my grandmother moved back from Florida, or my father stepped in, but somehow I returned to school to finish the year and I was never so grateful in all my life.

There are many events that shape our lives and forever change who we are. For me, this was one. When my mother became sick and lost her capacity for a time to walk, to talk and to do for herself, I never took another thing for granted again. In a way, it was a gift to both of us. We realized that time was not on our side. For Mom, she went on to earn two doctorates and became a celebrated engineer in both biophysics and naval architecture. For me, I learned that every day needed to be lived fully, because truly, you just never know what tomorrow is going to bring.

**It is hard to see Plan B as a gift,
yet perhaps it is given by the Universe?
Perhaps it is Divine?**

When things don't go our way, when things don't work out, it is certainly difficult to see it as an opportunity. When we see our loved ones suffer, perhaps they lose their jobs, or lose their abilities, when our children undergo setbacks and when our parents become ill, these are the most trying and mystifying of times. Yet, those times might be for a reason…

Change Your Story

When I first started practicing yoga many years ago, it seemed like I was the only one in the room with cellulite on my butt and kids in the kitchen. These days, many of my friends are catching up to me. They are experiencing the wakeup call of being older on the mat. In some ways, it is a lovely bird song to the soul. It makes touching your toes new again, every day you can. I don't really need the thrill of say, putting one foot behind my head and standing on my hands while breathing a six-count breath to make it a good day. (Although doing it is pretty thrilling, I might add.) Just being alive another day is such an incredible gift.

If the ultimate Plan B is to age, then the gift is that we realize we are running out of time.

Death wakes us up to our term limits.

If there are days on my mat where I don't want to try a pose, I remind myself I will be even older tomorrow. Better try now while I'm young! The same goes for telling people that I love them. Now might be a good time. Approaching the second half of my life is a chance to live better, wiser and stronger. I am more aware. I feel more connected. I am motivated by a huge, indescribable force, which in turn, inspires me to inspire others.

Yoga has shown me that I am who I am, and this is where I am supposed to be. For a girl who once moved so often that she had to keep her address written on a piece of paper pinned inside her blouse, I now feel safe and sound whenever I roll out my mat. It feels good to be home.

I have arrived and I'm ready to write a new ending to my story. Each of us has a story. Some of the chapters are written by us, by the decisions and choices we made; some of the chapters are written by the Universe and the stuff that happens. What we don't realize right away is that we can change our story at any time.

There is a part of the Divine that lives inside us, which we can cultivate and grow. We can play big, instead of small. Instead of reacting and running around like mad, we can slow down and see the amazing, extraordinary gift in the moment. We can listen more carefully to the pulsating hum within and without. We can surrender being the doer of all things, and let the Universe do for us. We can ride along in the currents of Grace and see where life takes us.

I am powered by Grace and inspired by life.

In fact, right about now, I might go home and make my family dinner! When the Harvard professor and philosopher Ram Dass asked his guru how he might reach enlightenment, his teacher replied, "Feed everyone." I am truly ready. My *dharma* is the duty I have now: to feed my family. I might even use the Cuisinart that's been sitting in the cupboard for twenty-five years. I think I'll give it a try. Nothing would make me happier than being with the ones I love. Not even a perfect Handstand. I have arrived … and I am home.

A Lesson From the Mat

Ten Reasons Why I Practice:

1. It beats the hell out of making dinner (until now).
2. It keeps me mentally, physically and spiritually engaged.
3. It helps me remember the light in my heart.
4. It helps me shut up and listen.
5. It reminds me that in my flaws are the seeds of my brilliance.
6. It reminds me that everything that holds me back can set me free.
7. It gives me a nice(r) butt. (Let's be honest.)
8. It is a creative outlet in my life.
9. It wakes me up, again and again, everyday.
10. I realize that wherever I am, I have arrived.

A Lesson From the Mat

How to Know If You Are NOT a Yogi (Yet):

- You think your practice is better than the person next to you.
- You think your practice is worse than the person next to you.
- Your clothes are super-cute, but you are kind of mean.
- You make the finger *mudra* of connecting Pointer to Thumbman on every pose. Meanwhile your back is killing you.
- You are still whining over stupid shit. (Come on, really? Is it ever going to end?)
- You see what's wrong with everything and everyone.
- If you think you are a yogi, then you may not be. But if you think you are never going to learn it all, then you probably are a yogi. Welcome to the path!

A Lesson From the Mat

How to Know If You ARE a Yogi (or Getting There):

- You look for the good. This is not a normal human response. You have to work at it. And if you come from New York, you have to work very hard at it.
- You operate from a place of love. No shit.
- You are trying to make peace with the past and with the people who have done you harm. You realize that everyone was trying to do their best, at that moment, and you forgive them. This is so hard, it's ridiculous. The yoga begins when you want to kill someone, and you don't. Or, as the *Bhagavad Gita* teaches us, you don't want to kill someone, and you must. Yoga *not* easy.
- You keep Patanjali's *Eight Limbed Path* on the top shelf of your moral pantry. Particularly *Ahimsa*— Do No Harm. The Ten Commandments are also a useful guide. And all that stuff your mother told you years ago. But above all else, try to do no harm.
- You start to see your choice in everything that happens to you.
- You know you are afraid and you carry on anyway. If you don't poop your pants now and then, you probably aren't taking enough risks.
- When you accept your shortcomings as your strengths, and your strengths as your possible

weaknesses, and you still love the whole stinking package, then you are a yogi. The same goes for the people in your life.

In every possible way, you try to leave the world a better place.

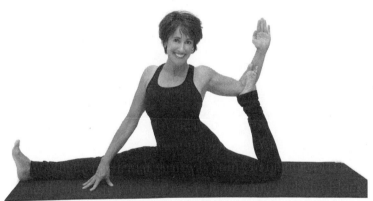

I have finally "arrived" at my dream pose, *Hanumanasana*.

Afterword

My Cuisinart is broken. Could it be a sign from the Universe?

I'm telling you:

I can't make this stuff up!

The Divine is everywhere.

After Afterword

My husband bought me a new Cuisinart.

Apparently, they are bigger than they used to be and now to store it I might need a new house or at least a new kitchen. The Universe is absolutely giving me a sign. I should forget about dinner and get back on my mat.

I am going to shut up now. Seriously. I know when to listen instead.

I Wish For You an Epic Fail

Believe you can and you are halfway there.
~ Theodore Roosevelt

If you've made it to the epilogue, I presume you know that I was divorced, flat broke and homeless. I had cancer, I was brutalized in a bathroom, and then like a phoenix, I rose from the ashes to become...wait for it...a soccer mom and a yoga teacher.

Nobody wants to hit bottom; however, if this happens to you, I highly recommend it. There is nothing like an epic fail to show you what you are made of.

The one episode I wish to revisit is how I went from flat broke to fabulous. It was not easy. And I certainly did not do it alone.

After my ex-husband left, with the wife of the former assistant city editor of the local newspaper, with all of our things including the car, with my dignity and my self-esteem, and lastly with the illusion of our happy marriage now completely blown apart, I was pretty scared.

I had my cocker spaniel and the toolbox my mother had given me. I had the dishes. I had a carful of things, but no car. I did not have a job, because I had given notice and the company had already filled the position. I was in Ohio, one thousand miles from home, and no idea where I was going to go.

Honestly, I did not even have the money for a bus ticket home.

But here is the thing about hitting bottom—you know which way is up. Having nothing makes you humble enough to ask for help. So I called my lawyer and said, "I do not have a job so I don't know if I can pay you." Miraculously, he got my job back.

I told a friend I did not have a car. He knew someone who would sell me a little white Honda with a sunroof and would look the other way on the loan papers. Thank you Jesus, God, Moses, Abraham, Buddha and Durga.

I walked into my old cubicle at the paper company, and said, "People, I have no place to live." My way back came in the form of Janet Blank, the marketing director. She said something like, "I know just how you feel."

An epic fail is something we can all relate to. I believe the ability to put one foot in front of the other is sometimes just about the bravest thing we can do.

Life and love are just like yoga.
We have to be willing to try over and over again,
until we get it right.

I moved in with Bob and Janet Blank of Dayton, Ohio. They opened their arms and hearts to me and my cocker spaniel. I was so thin from stress that Bob made his famous and fattening macaroni and cheese. Over a few months I got back to my normal weight and something of my normal self. My gratitude to them is boundless.

I had no intention of ever leaving the Blanks, but weeks turned into months and after nearly a year of hiding in their guest room, I decided it might be time to re-enter the real world. I tentatively took a lease on an apartment less than a mile away. Soon after that, my job would lead me back to New York.

Going Home, Again

There is nothing quite like returning home after an epic fail. You are changed. Of course, you may have the same hair or some of the same clothes, but your spirit will never be the same.

In my case, my epic fail set me free. I was no longer afraid of trying new things or taking on new challenges. I mean, what the hell? Right? Once you have lost everything, then you truly have nothing left to lose. It's not just a song lyric; it is life.

I accepted a job on Wall Street, I found an adorable apartment on the Upper West Side, and I dated with the vengeance of a woman looking for happiness.

So it seemed only logical to me that now that I was getting back on my feet and trying new things, that I should learn how to dance Hip Hop, next to perhaps taking singing lessons. For if there are two injustices in my life, it is that I cannot dance or sing.

Learning to Dance

My being a dancer is sort of like a five-foot person wanting to play in the NBA. As dreams go, it was a big one. But I had nothing after my epic fail, not even pride. I figured, as long as I'm having a giant Mulligan in my life, I might as well try dancing.

There were plenty of options to become a dancing fool so I enrolled at a school on the West Side. I started with the Fox Trot and the Waltz, and then I enrolled in Hip Hop.

At first, it was horrible. I was Lucille Ball going in the wrong direction. If the class was going up, I was going down. Left meant right. Forward meant backward.

My Roger Rabbit should have been euthanized.

But then I realized, of course I was going to be horrible at this. I can't dance! I have no rhythm. I have the attention span of a flea. I can't memorize the routines!

And that's when I became an okay dancer. In yoga we know that if we let go of expectations we will have a better chance at doing the pose. In dance it was the same. Once I had no expectations, it enabled me to dance (sort of). The school had a recital one evening and I invited Dad to watch. Afterwards he said, "You are better now than when you were little." Progress!

My pinnacle moment came when there was a Hip Hop singer looking for dancers for his new video. The school invited all interested students to try out. I wanted to do it.

Is that insane? I was a thirty-year-old klutz trying to be in a Hip Hop video. But here is the thing: no matter what happened it couldn't be as bad as being unloved, flat broke and homeless.

So I went. Marky Mark (Yes, *that* Marky Mark Wahlberg) sat on a chair. We were shown a routine to do on a diagonal across the room. All the girls jumped and twirled across the floor. When it was my turn, I pasted on my face the biggest smile you ever saw and leapt my way to the other side.

It was kind of a disaster.

But it didn't matter. I was elated. This was the most fun I'd had post-divorce. I didn't just leap across a room; I soared across a great divide of BEF (Before Epic Fail) to AEF (After Epic Fail). And I knew that if I could cross that room, then I could conquer anything in my path.

An epic fail will set you free. I highly recommend it.

Whatever life brings to you, do not be afraid to fail. For my next act, after journalist, high tech sales, racehorse rider, soccer mom and yogi, I think I'm going to try singing lessons. After all, I could not possibly be worse at it than I am now.

Acknowledgements

Life changes all the time and it is up to us to find our footing in a new world. For this edition, I have many teachers I need to thank, but I can't leave out Amy Ippoliti for lighting the way; Chris Muchow, my teacher in times past; Desiree Rumbaugh; and Christina Sell, who made me an "Asana Junkie." I have nothing but love for my yoga BFFs Jane Burdette and Michelle Weller, who traveled with me, practiced with me, and reminded me that we never walk alone.

Thank you to my photographers—Shannon Hedlund, who documented the early days on the mat, and Kimberly Benfield, who added a few updated views for this edition. Our practice progresses millimeter by millimeter.

Thank you to Hohm Press for seeing the potential in *Finding More on the Mat* and giving it this second chance. Gratitude to my editor Rabia Tredeau who made this second edition pitch perfect; and to Judith Briles, my first publishing editor, who taught me to dream big. Thanks, lady. Nick Zelinger, you are also in my heart for bringing my story to the printed page with so much flair.

Deep appreciation to my students as you encouraged me to write the themes I explain in the room. Thank you so much for your laughter through the tears!

Most of all, I want to thank my steadfast husband, Mike, and our sons Sam and Teddy. When I wanted to quit in the enormity of running a household, driving carpools, teaching yoga, and writing a book, you never let me.

Lastly, I want to acknowledge my Mom and Dad for giving me incredibly good genes and always doing your best. I think you are the most auspicious parents a yogi could have. For a girl who doesn't necessarily believe in luck, I am a very lucky girl.

Appendix A

The Yoga Sutras of Patanjali

*T*he *Yoga Sutras of Patanjali* were written almost 200 years ago. Patanjali's *sutras*, [aphorisms] focus on attaining the realization of the self. Here are his Ten Commandments, yogi-style:

Yamas, **the five universal moral restraints:**
- *Ahimsa* – non-violence, non-judgment, not harming
- *Satya* – truthfulness and honesty
- *Asteya* – not stealing
- *Brachmacharya* – chaste living (celibacy) or marital fidelity
- *Aparigraha* – non-hoarding, non-grasping, non-acceptance of gifts, being without possessions

Niyamas, **the five individual self-observances:**
- *Sauca* – cleanliness and purity
- *Santosa* – contentment
- *Tapas* – a burning desire for studentship and wisdom
- *Svadhyaya* – self study
- *Isvara Pranidhana* – devotion to a higher power, the Divine

Questions for Book Clubs

Finding More on the Mat: How I Grew Better, Wiser and Stronger Through Yoga is a 100% mostly true, often hilarious, sometimes sad, and always inspiring account of one woman's journey through life so far.

Suggested Discussion Topics:

- Michelle went from an accidental yogi to going all the way down the rabbit hole into yoga obsession. In what ways has something you've been passionate about in your life made you happier or more vibrant?

- *Finding More* is a story about *dharma,* or discovering what it is we are supposed to do in life. In what ways has your *dharma* changed over the years? Are you better off doing your *dharma*? What does it mean to do someone else's *dharma*?

- At the end of the book (spoiler alert!) Michelle decides that her true *dharma* at the moment isn't being on the mat, but making dinner for her family. In what ways is your *dharma* uncomfortable? Is doing your *dharma* supposed to be easy?

- One key point of yoga is to leave the world a little bit better than you found it. Explain how you do this, even if you don't practice yoga.

- When eating animal protein, you may also be eating its *karma*, so if they suffered terribly or was raised in an inhumane way, you will be eating the animal's stress hormones, fear and anger. What do you think of this concept?

- There are many ways to eat that reduce the carbon footprint and take care of our planet. Do you consider these things when making dinner?

- Michelle's tragic mishap as a young girl came back to haunt her in the form of a stuck shoulder as an adult. In what ways does the past haunt you today? Do you carry these things in your body? Has yoga improved this for you?

- Yoga has become a billion dollar business of celebrity and multinational corporations. In *Finding More*, Michelle's local teachers were responsible for most of her practice. If you practice yoga, how has your local teacher influenced your life?

- The story about setting the turtles free in Chapter 17 is about having to choose what is right even if it may be wrong or against the law. Has this ever happened to you? When is doing the right thing the most difficult? What makes it better?

- The message of the dedication, is "Always be exactly who you are." In what ways is it easier being your authentic and true self rather than hiding?

Recommended Reading

Baptiste, Baron. *Journey into Power*, NY: Simon & Schuster/ Fireside, 2003.

Chödrön, Pema. *When Things Fall Apart: Heart Advice for Difficult Times*. Boston, Mass.: Shambhala Publications, 1997.

Feuerstein, Georg, PhD. *The Yoga Tradition: Its History, Literature, Philosophy and Practice*. Chino Valley, AZ: Hohm Press, 1998.

Iyenger, B.K.S. *Light on Yoga: Yoga Dipika*. (1966) Revised Edition, NY: Pantheon/Random House/Schocken Books, 1995.

_____. *Light on the Yoga Sutras of Patanjali*. NY: Harper Collins/ Thorsons Publishers, New Edition, 2002.

Levine, Suzanne Braun. *Fifty is the New Fifty: Ten Life Lessons for Women in Second Adulthood*. NY: Penguin Group, Viking Press, 2009.

Mitchell, Stephen. *Bhagavad Gita: A New Translation*, NY: Crown/ Random House/Three Rivers Press, 2002.

Pennybacker, Minday. *Do One Green Thing: Saving the Earth Through Simple, Everyday Choices*. NY: St. Martin's Press/ Thomas Dunne Books, 2010.

Scaravelli, Vanda. *Awakening the Spine: The Stress-Free New Yoga that Works With the Body to Restore Health, Vitality and Energy*. CA: HarperSanFrancisco, 1991.

Sell, Christina. *Yoga from the Inside Out: Making Peace With Your Body Through Yoga*, Chino Valley, AZ: Hohm Press, 2003.

_____. *My Body is a Temple: Yoga as a Path to Wholeness*, Chino Valley, AZ: Hohm Press, 2011.

Finding "More" by the Chapter

Index

Index

Index

Index

OTHER YOGA TITLES OF INTEREST FROM HOHM PRESS

THE YOGA TRADITION
Its History, Literature, Philosophy and Practice
by Georg Feuerstein, Ph.D.
Foreword by Subhash Kak, Ph.D.

A complete overview of the great yogic traditions: Raja Yoga, Hatha Yoga, Jnana Yoga, Bhakti Yoga, Karma Yoga, Tantra Yoga, Kundalini Yoga, Mantra Yoga and many other lesser known forms. Includes translations of over twenty famous yoga treatises, including the *Yoga Sutra* of Patanjali, and a first-time translation of the *Goraksha Paddhati*, an ancient Hatha Yoga text. Covers all aspects of Hindu, Buddhist, Jaina and Sikh Yoga. This book is a necessary and unique reference work for all students and scholars of yoga from the foremost writer on yoga today.

Paper; 544 pages, over 200 illustrations; $29.95
ISBN: 978-1-890772-18-5
Yoga / Spirituality/ Eastern Philosophy

• • •

YOGA MORALITY
Ancient Teachings at a Time of Global Crisis
by Georg Feuerstein, Ph.D.

This book is a hard-hitting critique of the media hype surrounding yoga, and an exploration of yogic philosophy and practice to discover what it *really* means to be a mature and moral person. "It is impossible to be a good yogi or yogini without also being a morally mature individual," writes internationally known yoga authority and author, Georg Feuerstein. *Yoga Morality* looks at our present world situation primarily from the viewpoint of a spiritually committed person, especially a practitioner of yoga. It addresses the question: How are we to live consciously, responsibly, authentically, and without fear in the midst of mounting global crises?

Paper; 320 pages; $19.95   ISBN: 978-1-890772-66-6
Yoga / Religious Studies

To Order: call 1-800-381-2700. Visit our website, www.hohmpress.com

OTHER YOGA TITLES OF INTEREST FROM HOHM PRESS

MY BODY IS A TEMPLE
Yoga As a Path to Wholeness
by Christina Sell

With the freshness of a memoir, author and yoga teacher Christina Sell draws upon her first visit to an extraordinary temple in southern India to present basic principles of yoga. Beyond the ordinary aims of yoga as a means of stretching and strengthening, or even for being happier or more centered, *My Body is a Temple* is an instruction manual for dedicating oneself to a life of the spirit, in and through the vehicle of the human body. The body as a temple is a common metaphor within many spiritual traditions. In this book, Christina Sell delves into the "how" and "why" of this widely accepted comparison.

Paper; 248 pages; $16.95   ISBN: 978-1-935387-19-0
Yoga / Spirituality

• • •

YOGA FROM THE INSIDE OUT
Making Peace With Your Body Through Yoga
by Christina Sell

This is a book about Yoga and body image. More specifically, it is about Yoga and the issues of addiction, lack of self-love, and spiritual practice. Too many of us approach the practice of Yoga as another way to discipline the body without the inner softness necessary to be transformed by it. Author Christina Sell, a long-time student of Yoga and a master teacher, guides readers through a basic course in learning to accept *what is*, listen to the heart, and use the practice to deepen one's spiritual life.

Paper; 176 pages; $14.95   ISBN: 978-890772-32-1
Yoga / Body-Mind-Spirit

To Order: call 1-800-381-2700. Visit our website, www.hohmpress.com

OTHER YOGA TITLES OF INTEREST FROM HOHM PRESS

THE MATRIX OF YOGA
Teachings, Principles and Questions
by Georg Feuerstein and Brenda Feuerstein

This book offers novice yoga practitioners a solid foundation on which to begin or build their personal practice. Written by two highly respected yoga teachers and scholars in the West—Georg Feuerstein and his wife Brenda Feuerstein—the book will also augment yoga teacher trainings, and provide current yoga teachers with an invaluable text to use with or recommend to their new students. This reader-friendly handbook contains short essays that cover basic principles: the meaning of yoga, yoga practice, the types of yoga, and the deeper commitment and levels. In Part Two, the authors address thirty of the most widely asked questions by newcomers to the lifestyle and philosophy of this path.

Paper; 144 pages; $15.95   ISBN: 978-1-935387-47-3
Yoga / Religious Studies

• • •

THE MAKING OF A YOGA MASTER
A Seeker's Transformation
by Suhas Tambe

This book reveals the original sequence of Patanjali's sutras, which has been hidden for generations. Far more than an instruction manual, this book is also about one seeker's progression. The author, who began his search entrenched in materialism (he is an accountant with an MBA working in IT), was "transformed" into a devoted yoga practitioner. This path thoroughly changed his life's priorities, evolved his purpose, and dissolved old habits in a way that will be inspiring to many. "Yoga not just entered my life," he writes, "but now, it is my life." The Making of a Yoga Master marries the philosophy of yoga with clear "how-to" instructions and practical guidelines.

Paper; 416 pages; $24.95   ISBN: 978-1-935387-24-4
Yoga / Spirituality

To Order: call 1-800-381-2700. Visit our website, www.hohmpress.com

About the Author

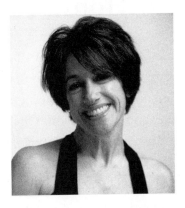

Michelle Berman Marchildon is The Yogi Muse. She's an internationally known author, columnist, yoga teacher and former executive who left the glamour of a corporate job to raise her family. In the midst of all that excitement, she found time to go upside down on her yoga mat.

Michelle is an award-winning journalist having won AP, UPI and Scripps Howard writing honors, and an alumnus of the Columbia Graduate School of Journalism. She is a Featured Columnist for *Elephant Journal*, a Columnist for *Origin* and *Mantra Yoga and Health* magazine, an ambassador for *Teachasana*, and a contributor to other yoga media.

For yoga teachers, Michelle wrote the bestselling book: *Theme Weaver: Connect the Power of Inspiration to Teaching Yoga*, which explains how to use a theme in yoga classes. She is an E-RYT 500 Hatha teacher in Denver, Colorado. Michelle is available for workshops and readings, especially if it gets her out of making dinner. Contact her through: www.YogiMuse.com

About Hohm Press

HOHM PRESS is committed to publishing books that provide readers with alternatives to the materialistic values of the current culture, and promote self-awareness, the recognition of interdependence, and compassion. Our subject areas include parenting, transpersonal psychology, religious studies, women's studies, the arts and poetry.

Hohm Press, PO Box 4410, Chino Valley, Arizona, 86323; USA; 800-381-2700, or 928-636-3331; email: hppublisher@ cableone.net

Visit our website at www.hohmpress.com